OXFORD MEDICAL PUBLICATIONS

BIOLOGICAL RHYTHMS AND EXERCISE

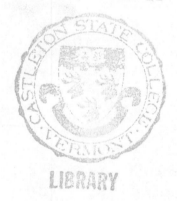

BIOLOGICAL RHYTHMS AND EXERCISE

T. REILLY, G. ATKINSON, AND J. WATERHOUSE

Centre for Sport and Exercise Sciences
School of Human Sciences
Liverpool John Moores University
Mountford Building
Byrom Street
Liverpool L3 3AF

OXFORD NEW YORK TOKYO

OXFORD UNIVERSITY PRESS

1997

Oxford University Press, Walton Street, Oxford OX2 6DP
Oxford   New York
Athens   Auckland   Bangkok   Bombay
Calcutta   Cape   Town   Dar es Salaam   Delhi
Florence   Hong Kong   Istanbul   Karachi
Kuala   Lampur   Madras   Madrid   Melbourne
Mexico   City   Nairobi   Paris   Singapore
Taipei   Tokyo   Toronto
and associated companies in
Berlin   Ibadan

Oxford is a trade mark of Oxford University Press

Published in the United States
by Oxford University Press Inc., New York

© T. Reilly, G. Atkinson and J. Waterhouse, 1997

A catalogue record for this book is available from the British Library

Library of Congress Cataloging in Publication Data
(Data Applied for)

ISBN 0 19 262525 X (h/b)
ISBN 0 19 262524 1 (p/b)

Typeset by Hewer Text Composition Services, Edinburgh
Printed in Great Britain by
Bookcraft Ltd, Midsomer Norton, Nr Bath

Preface

This text is focused on the relations between biological rhythms and exercise. Existence of biological rhythms is now reflected in the acknowledgement of chronobiology as a valid scientific field. Information on human biological rhythms has been applied to various occupational and ergonomics contexts over the last couple of decades, including aviation, travel, and other industries. Awareness of the significance of rhythmic biological changes is now realized in sports and exercise settings. This is manifested in the requests for counselling of national sports teams on travel plans, individual women athletes about menstrual status and the regular appearance of short reviews on these subjects in sports medicine periodicals. Modules on 'biological rhythms' are incorporated into the programmes of undergraduate and post-graduate courses in sports science and in sports medicine. Whilst there has been texts written on 'women athletes' which have incorporated a discussion of exercise and the menstrual cycle, there has been no text concerned with circadian rhythms and exercise nor on an integration of biological rhythms of various cycle lengths into an exercise context.

The aims of this text are to:

i)   provide a comprehensive account of biological rhythms and apply this to a sport and exercise setting;
ii) detail the effect of circadian rhythms on human performance in general and on responses to exercise in particular;
iii) integrate knowledge about circadian rhythms and exercise into a systematic treatment of the relations between biological rhythms, sport performance and training;
iv) outline the consequences of disrupting normal circadian rhythms, either by loss of sleep, crossing multiple time-zones or by working nocturnal shifts.
v)   consider in a systematic manner the impact that rhythms of various cycle lengths have for sport and exercise practitioners;
vi) synthesize the research information from chronobiology laboratories for students, researchers, and practitioners of sport.

The book is suitable for students, research, and academic staff in Universities and Colleges of Further Education where there is an interest in Sports Science or the application of biological rhythms to sport and exercise. It will be of use also to coaches and athletes wishing to gain detailed information on this aspect of training and preparation for sports events. The material is relevant to personnel engaged in fitness assessments and to sports medical staff concerned with evaluating individual responses to exercise.

The book is organized so that the principles of chronobiology are presented before the applications to sport and exercise are described. The opening chapter provides a comprehensive description of biological rhythms and their scientific foundation. This is followed by an outline of physiological rhythms at rest which have potential impacts on exercise contexts. Circadian rhythms in mental performance are then described. The chapter on rhythms in sport performance includes physiological, physical and subjective responses to exercise. The sleep-wakefulness cycle is considered in the next chapter in which sleep processes are explained and the consequences of sleep loss discussed. The desynchronization of circadian rhythms resulting from crossing multiple time-zones is the subject of Chapter 6. The consequences of disturbing circadian rhythms are detailed for travelling athletes and nocturnal shiftwork respectively in the next two chapters. Rhythms with longer cycles, circamensal (monthly) and circannual (season) are covered in Chapters 9 and 10. The text culminates in an exposition of research methodology in chronobiology to present readers with an insight into the nuances of studying biological rhythms.

In each of the chapters we have attempted to translate the results of a vast amount of studies on biological rhythms into applications for sport and human performance. The references cited are indicative of research work completed rather than a complete list of experimental reports. The 'further reading' recommended with each chapter gives readers an opportunity to extend their studies on the subject. In these ways we hope that our own knowledge about biological rhythms is transmitted to the reader and that this text forms a starting point for further study.

Liverpool   T.R.
April 1996   G.A.
                                                                                                       J.W.

Contents

1
Introduction to chronobiology

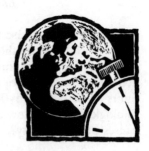

1.1 Environmental and biological rhythmicity

Evolution has resulted in humans being anatomically, physiologically, and behaviourally adjusted to their environment. Thus, they show adaptation to an upright posture, they control their body temperature in spite of large swings in ambient temperature, and they control the composition of their plasma in spite of the dehydrating effects of the atmosphere and taking in food and drink discontinuously. Ecologically, humans have responded to environmental demands, whether these be due to gravity, temperature or dehydration. Another influence – that of time – is equally important, and humans, like all other living organisms, have also responded to the changes produced by time in their bodies.

There can be no doubt that the daily, or circadian, rhythms due to the alternation of day and night would have influenced our cave-dwelling ancestors. Even though the use of artificial lighting and of darkened bedrooms has given civilized societies considerable independence from natural daylight, it is clear that we still consider ourselves as diurnal creatures – active in the daytime, asleep at night – and that most of society's infrastructure reflects this.

Other environmental rhythms are important, though more so to species other than humans. Annual rhythms, particularly at high latitudes, and tidal rhythms can be very powerful influences. Tidal rhythms are complex. Their basic period is 12.4 h, but the tides also interact with the sun's gravitational forces to produce the spring and neap tides, which are about 15 days apart. Both these environmental rhythms are reflected in biological cycles in living organisms.

Other rhythms are present in humans and their period cannot always be obviously related to an environmental influence. Menstrual cycles, with a length averaging 28 days, and weekly cycles (e.g. in waking time) are known as infradian rhythms. By contrast, there is a whole range of ultradian rhythms with periods of less than about 21 h. The periods of these rhythms range from a fraction of a second (e.g. alpha-, theta-, and delta-wave activity in the brain) through a second or more (e.g. heart rate, respiratory frequency), to an hour or more (e.g. types of sleep, activity and rest in neonates, release of pituitary hormones into the bloodstream).

Biological rhythms are not only produced as a direct effect of the environment. There are alternative possibilities. First, they can result from a behavioural response to the environment, such as a change in sleep and activity produced by the light–dark cycle, or a rhythm of urine production secondary to one of fluid intake. Second, rhythmicity can result from the actions of feedback loops that control biological variables within narrow limits. Third, the rhythm might originate from some form of internal 'biological clock'. How could a distinction be drawn between these possible causes of rhythmicity?

1.1.1 Exogenous and endogenous rhythms

Those rhythms that are produced by pre-existing ones in the environment are easily removed by studying an individual in an environment from which the rhythmic influence has been removed, or where the rhythmic influence has been changed. By using the first protocol, it has been shown that many seasonal rhythms – or example, those of migratory restlessness, mating behaviour in many mammals, hibernation, leaf abscission and spring flowering – are all lost in an environment in which the amount of daylight per 24 hours does not change. If, instead, the time cues in the environment are changed, then the rhythms observed in the body also change immediately and stay in phase with the external cues. Examples in humans are: the ultradian rhythms in a nursing mother (due to her baby's periodic demand for food); ultradian rhythms in plasma insulin (due to food intake); the secretion of growth hormone (GH) in the daytime in a nightworker (because the sleep–activity cycle has been inverted); the daily rhythm of length of the spinal column (because it lengthens whenever an individual unloads it by lying down to sleep); the weekly rhythm in the total volume of urine produced in 24 hours (if the individual drinks more at the weekend); and the yearly rhythm in suntan (even if it necessitates a summer holiday abroad!). In all these cases, since the timing of the rhythms (their phase and frequency) is determined by external factors, the rhythms are called exogenous. Most seasonal rhythms are strongly exogenous and these will be considered in Chapter 10.

Biological rhythms, however, do not always follow an external influence. The failure of rhythms in humans to follow imposed time cues can be demonstrated in several ways similar to those above. Thus, such rhythms would continue with a normal frequency and timing on a constant routine (i.e. one in which the subject stays awake, eats frequently and snacks regularly, and maintains a constant activity in an environment of unchanging temperature and lighting), and in one in which external time cues were changed. Such changes – as applied to circadian rhythms – can be brought about by placing individuals in another time-zone, by requiring them to invert their sleep–activity schedule (e.g. during nightwork) or to live a normal lifestyle but based on a non-24-hour 'day', such as one lasting 21 or 28 hours.

For ultradian or infradian rhythms, the same principles are involved, but the time cues that would need to be manipulated have different periods (e.g. changes in mealtimes or seasonal fluctuations in lighting or temperature). Since such rhythms appear to originate from inside the body, they are therefore called endogenous.

Since many rhythms are a mixture of endogenous and exogenous components, the experiments just described can be more complex to interpret. For example, after a shift in habits or when on a non-24-hour imposed 'day', an individual's rhythms might show both an unchanged component – reflecting the endogenous component – and a changed component (reflecting the altered lifestyle – the exogenous component). Also, in a time-free environment, a rhythm might not disappear, but instead get smaller in amplitude.

The example of the circadian rhythm of body temperature will make this clear. Figure 1.1 shows the normal appearance of this rhythm and its appearance after removal of the exogenous component, due to the sleep–activity cycle and daytime meals. The full line shows the daily rhythm due to the combined endogenous and exogenous components, whereas the dashed line represents the endogenous (clock) component in the absence of any rhythmic environment and lifestyle. The difference between the two curves is due to the exogenous component alone. This figure not only shows the two components clearly, but also indicates that normally these two components are in phase and so accentuate each other.

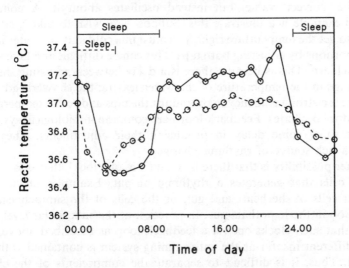

Fig. 1.1 Mean circadian changes in rectal temperature measured hourly in eight subjects living a normal existence (full line), and in the same subjects given a constant routine of being woken at 04:00 and spending the subsequent 24 hours awake in a constant light and taking hourly small identical snacks (dashed line) (Minors and Waterhouse 1981).

1.1.2 Causes of endogenous rhythms

Establishing that a rhythm originates inside the body – or at least has a component that is endogenous – does not distinguish between the different causes of this oscillation. Two possible explanations are:

1. There is some sort of control loop which shows oscillation.
2. There is a structure inside the body that acts like a clock.

Feedback loops are the common way in which the body controls variables within narrow limits, as must be achieved in health. The control of body temperature provides an illustration of this process. If body temperature rises, then mechanisms that promote heat loss (cutaneous vasodilatation, sweating) are initiated; the result of these changes is that body temperature falls to a set value and the error has been corrected. Similarly, if body temperature starts to fall, then a different set of mechanisms (shivering, constriction of blood vessels to the skin) is set in motion to raise body temperature. The system can be described in control-theory terms as a temperature change which initiates compensatory mechanisms which oppose the temperature change.

It can be seen from this why such a control mechanism is called a feedback loop. Such a feedback loop takes time to exert its effect, as a result of which the variable that is being controlled (in this case, body temperature) does not stay at the 'correct' value, but instead oscillates about it. A common household example will illustrate this. Suppose you wish to take a shower and that, to get the temperature right, you must mix cold and hot water in the right proportions by adjusting both taps. This can be difficult and take some while to achieve. This is because there is a delay between adjusting the tap and a change in the temperature of the water leaving the showerhead; as a result there is a strong tendency to overadjust the taps and so the temperature of the mixture oscillates. Feedback loops are common in biological systems, and most show some delay in producing their adjustments. They are therefore a rich source of rhythmic change.

The other possibility is that there is some form of 'clock', that is, a cell or group of cells that generates a rhythmic output. Examples include the pacemaker cells of the heart and gut, or the cells of the suprachiasmatic nuclei (SCN) in the hypothalamus. In practice, at the subcellular level, it is probable that such clocks act via a feedback loop as described above, but they are different insofar as the entire timing system is contained within a single cell. Thus, it is difficult to separate the components of the clock, whereas, in the feedback loops described above, the components are often in separate groups of cells or even in different parts of the body. As a result of this difference in scale, it is comparatively easy to separate the components of a feedback loop and so stop the rhythm.

We will illustrate these ideas by referring in more detail to respiration rhythm and heart rate. These are both examples of ultradian rhythms, which have a period of less than 21 h and are commonly found in the body.

Respiration rhythm originates from two groups of cells that show reciprocal inhibition and self-excitation. Simply explained, one group of cells (the inspiratory centre) starts firing; this causes them to excite themselves and their agonists and to stimulate inspiration. After a while, and for several reasons, the firing rate of this group of cells then begins to decline. This will remove inhibition from the opponent group of cells (the expiratory centre), which will therefore begin to fire. This then causes the expiratory cells to stimulate themselves, but to inhibit their antagonists in the inspiratory centre, so promoting expiration. After a while, the expiratory cells will fatigue, the inspiratory centre will begin to fire, and the process begins again.

With regard to heart rate, the isolated denervated heart will continue to beat spontaneously, due to a rhythmic, electrical discharge of pacemaker cells in the sinoatrial node. These cells have unstable membrane potentials caused by linked changes in the degree of opening and closing of different membrane channels. After depolarizing to threshold, an action potential is initiated. Since the cells of the heart behave as an electrical syncytium, a wave of electrical activity passes through the heart muscle causing muscle contraction. When the action potential is over, the membrane channels are reset to their original state and the process recommences spontaneously.

The respiratory rhythm stops if either the inspiratory or expiratory centre is isolated. That is, it is the interaction or feedback between the two that is the fundamental cause of the rhythmicity. By contrast, single cells of the heart pacemaker continue to depolarize rhythmically, even if they are separated from the rest of the heart, so that there is no feedback between contraction of the heart muscle and the activity of the pacemaker cell. This difference leads us to another way of distinguishing between the two means of generating rhythmicity. Since, in the case of the heartbeat, the rhythm comes from a group of cells acting independently of the contraction processes they initiate, once the disturbance is over, the heartbeat will continue with a timing determined by the pacemaker cells and be independent of the time-course of the disrupting influence. By contrast, if the process of breathing is disturbed then, after removal of the disturbance, the system resumes rhythmicity, but from the point in the cycle at which the disturbance exerted its effect.

The current view is that the endogenous component of circadian rhythmicity originates from a 'bodyclock' (see below), and that many rhythms with longer (infradian) or shorter (ultradian) periods are due to feedback loops. For many rhythms in hormone secretion, it appears that there are two frequencies of rhythm – ultradian and circadian – and that they are caused by different mechanisms. Thus, the ultradian rhythm is produced by neural networks that are believed to have properties similar to those causing rhythmicity in the respiratory system – some form of neurally mediated feedback loop. However, the circadian component derives from the circadian bodyclock.

Menstrual cycles (circamensal rhythms with a period of about 1 month) illustrate clearly the generation of rhythmicity due to a series of feedback loops and associated time delays between cause and effect. These will be described in Chapter 9.

Our main concern in the present book is circadian rhythms. It is some of the properties of these that we will now consider.

1.2 Some properties of body time

In order to study body time in more detail, time cues from the outside environment must be removed for at least several days so that the individual is completely free from such influences. In this way, it is argued, any rhythmicity that remains must come from within the individual – an endogenous component. This is known as a free-running experiment. Early experiments required individuals to stay in underground caves, while more recently, specially constructed isolation units have been used (Halberg *et al.* 1970; Wever 1979). Both types of experiment have shown that circadian rhythms continue in such environments; the timing of an individual's habits and rhythms, such as times of retiring or rising, of eating, or of minimum body temperature, do not become random with the passage of days or weeks.

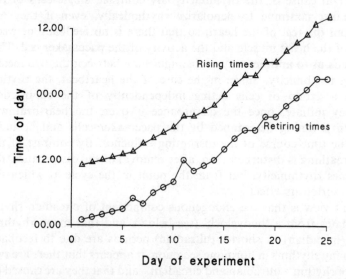

Fig. 1.2 Times of retiring and rising on successive occasions in an individual isolated from all knowledge of the passage of time in, a free-running experiment (Waterhouse *et al.* 1990).

However, the rhythm measured under free-running conditions does not last exactly 24 hours but is slightly longer, approximately 25 hours in humans (Fig. 1.2). For this reason, such a rhythm is called circadian (Latin: *circa*, about; *dies*, a day). The fact that the cycle length, or period, of the bodyclock differs from 24 h is very strong evidence for its origin being independent of the external environment and, indeed, being inside the body itself. This period of the bodyclock is called its free-running period.

Close inspection of Fig. 1.2 shows another important result. When the individual stayed awake longer than usual (e.g as on day 11), then the length of sleep was shorter than usual. This was because waking time was not delayed by as great an amount as the subject had stayed awake. This suggests that the length of sleep is not determined by the amount of prior wakefulness, but rather that waking tends to occur at a certain phase of the bodyclock – going to bed late means this point is reached after a shorter amount of sleep. The opposite applies if we go to bed earlier than usual (e.g. day 7 in Fig. 1.2) because it takes a longer time for the appropriate phase to be reached.

The fact that the bodyclock is a poor timekeeper (compared with solar time) threatens to undermine its usefulnes. In practice, however, the body-clock is adjusted to an exact 24-hour period by several rhythms from the environment and the individual's habits. These rhythms are called zeitgebers (German: *zeit*, time; *geber*, to give). For many animals, it is the alternation of light and darkness between day and night that acts as a zeitgeber. Indeed, this is acknowledged by our description of animals as 'nocturnal' or 'diurnal'. Other environmental influences, such as food availability and social cues, can also play a role, particularly in the interactions between parent and newborn offspring. In humans, natural lighting can adjust the bodyclock (as can artificial light of a sufficient intensity), but regular mealtimes, activity, and social influences are all effective to some degree also. These 'alternative' zeitgebers are likely to be the dominant ones for many people who are rarely exposed to natural light, particularly during the winter, or for the blind. In practice, it is most useful to consider all potential time cues as providing a 'zeitgeber package' that continually adjusts the bodyclock.

1.3 The site of the bodyclock

The site of the bodyclock has been the subject of much research, necessarily conducted upon animals. There is now a very large amount of data which points to the hypothalamic, paired, SCN as being a crucial part of the internal timing system. The main lines of evidence are the following (Minors and Waterhouse 1981, 1986):

1. The SCN show a circadian rhythm in the uptake of the nonmetabolized glucose analogue, 2-deoxy-D-glucose.

2. The firing rate of neurones in the SCN continues to show a circadian rhythm when the SCN cells have been separated from the rest of the central nervous system (CNS) by surgery. This indicates that the SCN cells are *not* rhythmic in (1) above because of a rhythmic neural input, such as from a clock elsewhere in the brain.

3. Slices of SCN incubated *in vitro* show circadian rhythms of neuronal firing frequency and release of neurotransmitter. This result removes the possibility that humoral factors accounted for the rhythm in (2) above.

4. Removal of the SCN leads to losses of circadian activity and drinking in animals. Such rhythmicity can be recovered if fetal hypothalamic cells from the germinal areas for the SCN are transplanted into the animal. Moreover, if material is used from a fetus with a mutant clock (i.e. an animal that, when adult, will show abnormally rapid or slow circadian rhythms), then the rhythm that develops in the host shows the mutant period (Ralph *et al.* 1990). This last finding indicates that the clock itself, that is, a structure able to generate a *particular* periodicity has been transplanted, rather than some structure able to produce a generalised rhythmicity.

1.3.1 The pineal gland – part of the bodyclock?

There is also evidence that the pineal gland, a structure in the roof of the midbrain which secretes the hormone melatonin, plays some part in generating and controlling body time. In birds and other animals which show seasonal rhythms, e.g. in migration or breeding, the pineal gland is an important link between changes in the external environment and the many biochemical and physiological changes they evoke. In humans, such seasonal changes appear to be far less important, but this additional link between rhythmicity in the environment and the body remains, and probably adds to the accuracy of timing of the bodyclock. Receptors for melatonin are present in the SCN and this would support the view that some functional connection exists. This evidence, and that summarized in the next section, lead to the current view that the SCN and pineal gland interact to form the bodyclock.

1.3.2 How zeitgebers work

The ways in which zeitgebers act also suggest that the SCN and pineal gland have complementary roles. An anatomical link between the retina and the SCN – the retinohypothalamic tract – has been found. This carries information about environmental lighting to the SCN. For example, it has been shown that a pulse of bright light given to hamsters kept in constant dark can adjust the bodyclock, with the amount and direction of adjustment depending upon the time when the bright light is given. A similar response has also been observed recently in humans (Minors *et al.*

1991). Bright light at the end of the night, just after the minimum body temperature has occurred (Fig. 1.1), tends to advance the bodyclock; bright light at the beginning of the night and just before the minimum temperature tends to delay it; and in the middle of the day, bright light has no effect. Melatonin is normally secreted in the late evening and at night and is suppressed by bright light. Ingestion of this hormone also appears to produce shifts of the bodyclock; evening doses advance it and morning doses delay it. In other words, melatonin secretion has the opposite effect to bright light and can be considered to act as a 'dark pulse', as far as adjusting the bodyclock is concerned (Lewy *et al.* 1992). In practice, bright light in the morning therefore advances the bodyclock, not only via the retinohypothalamic tract, but also because it suppresses melatonin secretion and so prevents the delay of the bodyclock that melatonin would normally produce at this time. Similarly, bright light in the evening delays the bodyclock by both mechanisms. As a result, the circadian bodyclock can be adjusted to an exact 24-hour period. The means by which social and physical activities and mealtimes might act as zeitgebers is less well known. Even so, this lack of information does not reduce the role they can play, and need not negate their value for promoting adjustment of the bodyclock to jetlag or shiftwork (Chapters 6 and 8).

1.4 The usefulness of circadian rhythms

What use is served by circadian rhythms? Briefly, they enable the effects upon the body of regular environmental changes to be predicted. They are therefore fundamentally different from control by feedback loops, where the response to changes in the body, produced by the environment, takes place after the event (Moore-Ede 1986). Thus, the actions of the bodyclock mean that plasma adrenaline concentration and body temperature both rise before waking, preparing us for the rigours of a new day, and fall in the evening, preparing us for relaxation and sleep. Such changes, produced by the bodyclock, are independent of the external environment. Of course, they can also be adjusted by feedback control when necessary.

There is a further link between the bodyclock and feedback loops. It appears that the output from the bodyclock can change the sensitivity and threshold of various elements in a feedback loop. For example, sweating and cutaneous vasodilatation are initiated at lower temperatures during the night than the day. As a result, the thermoregulatory system shows circadian variation, with body temperature being controlled at a lower value during the night than the day.

Clearly, this combination of the bodyclock and feedback loops enables an individual to prepare for predictable changes in the environment, as well as to respond to any unexpected changes. The body as a whole shows circadian rhythmicity because the major rhythmic outputs of the bodyclock, such as those of body temperature, the sympathetic nervous system, and plasma adrenaline and other hormones, exert their effects very widely.

1.5 Differences between individuals

As with any other biological variable, individuals are not identical when rhythms are considered. Such differences are caused by the amplitude of rhythms, the relative importance of exogenous and endogenous factors in causing them, details of the importance of different zeitgebers, and the phase or timing of different rhythms. The causes of such differences are seldom known in detail, but our different lifestyles, e.g. whether active or sedentary, whether concentrated in the earlier or later portions of the day, will all contribute to this variation. Internal factors also contribute. These arise because the bodyclock differs between individuals in its exact free-running period, in how accurately it responds to zeitgebers, and in the relative importance of the different zeitgebers.

Two differences affect our responses to abnormal sleep–activity schedules, namely after a time-zone transition and during nightwork (Chapters 6 and 8). These differences are age and how much of a morning-type (lark) or evening-type (owl) we are. The following questionnaire enables you to gain some idea of how much of a lark or owl you might be. The questionnaire is based on that by Horne and Ostberg (1976).

1. What time would you choose to get up if you were free to plan your day?
   A 05:00–06:00
   B 06:00–07:30
   C 07:30–10:00
   D 10:00–11:00
   E 11:00–12:00
2. You have some important business to attend to, for which you want to feel at the peak of your mental powers. When would you prefer this meeting to take place?
   A 08:00–10:00
   B 11:00–13:00
   C 15:00–17:00
   D 19:00–21:00
3. What time would you choose to go to bed if you were entirely free to plan your evening?
   A 20:00–21:00
   B 21:00–22:15
   C 22:15–00:30
   D 00:30–01:45
   E 01:45–03:00

4. A friend wishes to go jogging with you, and suggests starting at 07:00–08:00. How would you feel at this time?
   A On good form
   B On reasonable form
   C You would find it difficult
   D You would find it very difficult
5. You now have some physical work to do. At what time would you feel able to do it best?
   A 08:00–10:00
   B 11:00–13:00
   C 15:00–17:00
   D 19:00–21:00
6. You have to go to bed at 23:00. How would you feel?
   A Not at all tired, and unable to get to sleep quickly
   B Slightly tired, but unlikely to get to sleep
   C Fairly tired, and likely to get to sleep quickly
   D Very tired, and very likely to get to sleep quickly
7. When you have been up for half an hour on a normal working day, how do you feel?
   A Very tired
   B Fairly tired
   C Fairly refreshed
   D Very refreshed
8. At what time of the day do you feel best?
   A 08:00–10:00
   B 11:00–13:00
   C 15:00–17:00
   D 19:00–21:00
9. Another friend suggests jogging at 22:00–23:00. How would you now feel?
   A On good form
   B On reasonable form
   C You would find it difficult
   D You would find it very difficult

Now score the answers, and add up the points for the nine questions.

Q.1 A = 1	Q.2 A = 1	Q.3 A = 1
B = 2	B = 2	B = 2
C = 3	C = 3	C = 3
D = 4	D = 4	D = 4
E = 5		E = 5
Q.4 A = 1	Q.5 A = 1	Q.6 A = 4
B = 2	B = 2	B = 3
C = 3	C = 3	C = 2
D = 4	D = 4	D = 1
Q.7 A = 4	Q.8 A = 1	Q.9 A = 4
B = 3	B = 2	B = 3
C = 2	C = 3	C = 2
D = 1	D = 4	D = 1

The score can range from 9 to 38 and is interpreted as follows:

- 9–15 definitely a lark
- 16–20 moderately a lark
- 21–26 neither a lark nor an owl but intermediate in chronotype
- 27–31 moderately an owl
- 32–38 definitely an owl.

Most people score between 21–26, and are intermediate in type. As can be deduced from the questionnaire, larks or morning-types are keen to start the day early and to work hardest then. Their evening is spent preparing for sleep. Owls are the opposite; they prefer to go to bed and to get up late, and to work hardest later in the day.

Even though only a small proportion of the population (5%) is extreme in terms of being owls or larks, a larger proportion shows this trait to a lesser extent. They will have greater or lesser problems than 'intermediate' individuals in coping with morning-shifts, night-shifts, and longhaul flights.

It is not possible to say, in any particular case, if the cause is internal (the properties of the clock) or external (the lifestyle and zeitgebers). Often, the internal and external factors tend to reinforce each other when individuals are free to choose. Thus, those who, by virtue of their bodyclock, tend to be owls are more likely to work and be active later in the day, and to like to sleep late into the morning. Their chosen lifestyle will tend to exaggerate such traits. Problems might arise if, for example, larks have to work at night for extended periods of time, or owls have long stretches on morning-shifts.

1.6 The myth of biorhythms

It is unfortunate that the rhythms produced by the brain and described above are sometimes called 'biorhythms', because this term is also used to describe a nonscientific model. According to this model, there are three rhythms, with periods of 23, 28, and 33 days, that predetermine when we will have 'good' and 'bad' days. The three cycles are supposed to represent physical, emotional and intellectual abilities, respectively, and to have started their inexorable cycling when we were born. Scientifically, such a theory is untenable since, in its strongest form, it neither explains the origins of the rhythms, nor allows interindividual variation, nor includes the possibility of changes during an individual's lifetime. Nevertheless, it is reasonable to ask if it works, i.e. if it has predictive power.

All anecdotal and retrospective accounts are of course suspect, since only the 'hits' will be recorded by believers and 'misses' by sceptics. A scientific test would at least require individuals or observers to assess days as 'good' or 'bad' in ignorance of the predictions of biorhythm theory. This has been done only rarely and the results were not significantly different from chance (Klein and Wegman 1979). Investigations of the season's best performance of 610, elite, track and field athletes from Europe failed to show any influence of the computed 'biorhythms' on peak performances (Reilly *et al.* 1983). This does not mean that we do not have good and bad days – however they are assessed – but rather that these cannot be predicted reliably by the biorhythm theory.

1.7 Overview

When the human body is studied, many variables show rhythms with periods ranging from seconds to a year. These rhythms originate from either external sources (and so might be controlled) or from internal ones (and so are more difficult to adjust). Although the examples discussed so far might not appear to be directly relevant to sport, the following should be considered:

1. These rhythms might offset sports performance directly, or indirectly through for example, loss of motivation or lack of sleep.
2. Other aspects of sports performance, such as muscle strength or coordination, might also be rhythmic.
3. The slow adjustment of the bodyclock to a change in the sleep–activity schedule will be important to athletes travelling to sports meetings in distant parts of the world.

It is these possibilities that form the subject of the rest of the book. It must be admitted at the outset that only a small amount of research on rhythms has been done with sportsmen and sportswomen specifically in mind. However, much work has been performed on young healthy adults, the results of which can be applied to people for whom exercise is important.

Further reading

Moore-Ede, M., Sulzman, F., and Fuller, C. (1982). *The clocks that time us*. Harvard, Cambridge, MA, USA.
Waterhouse, J. (1994). Altered time. In *Human physiology* (ed. R. Case and J. Waterhouse), pp. 211–30 Oxford University Press.
Young, M. (1988). *The metronomic society*. Thames and Hudson, London.

References

Halberg, F., Reinberg, A., and Haus, E. (1970). Human biological rhythms during and after several months of isolation underground in natural caves. *Bull. Natl. Speleological Soc.*, **32**, 89–115.
Horne, J. and Ostberg, O. (1976). A self-assessment questionnaire to determine morningness–eveningness in human circadian rhythms. *Int. J. Chronobiol.*, **4**, 97–110.

Klein, K. and Wegman, H. (1979) Circadian rhythms in air operations. In *Sleep, wakefulness and circadian rhythm*, AGARD Lecture Series 105, NATO, Neuilly sur Seine, Section 10.

Lewy, A., Ahmed, S., Jackson, J., and Sack, R. (1992). Melatonin shifts human circadian rhythms according to a phase–response curve. *Chronobiol. Int.*, **9**, 380–92.

Minors, D. and Waterhouse, J. (1981). *Circadian rhythms and the human.* Wright, Bristol.

Minors, D. and Waterhouse, J. (1986). *Circadian rhythms and their mechanisms Experientia*, **42**, 1–13.

Minors, D., Waterhouse, J., and Wirz-Justice, A. (1991). A human phase–response curve to light. *Neurosci. Lett.*, **133**, 36–40.

Moore-Ede, M. (1986). Physiology of the circadian timing system: predictive versus reactive homeostasis. *Amer. J. Physiol.*, **250**, R737–R752.

Ralph, M., Foster, R., Davis, F., and Menaker, M. (1990). Transplanted suprachiasmatic nucleus determines circadian period. *Science*, **247**, 975–8.

Reilly, T., Young, K., and Seddon, R. (1983). Investigations of biorhythms in female athlete performance. *Appl. Ergonom.* **14**, 215–17.

Waterhouse, J., Minors, D., and Waterhouse, M. (1990). *Your body clock.* Oxford University Press.

Wever, R. (1979). *The circadian system of man.* Springer-Verlag, New York.

2
Physiological rhythms at rest

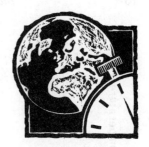

2.1 Introduction

The existence of physiological rhythms at rest must be taken into consideration by the exercise scientist. First, measurements at resting state should be controlled for the time of day to avoid potential misinterpretation later. Second, the time of day may influence the preparedness of the subject for submaximal and maximal exercise performance. As a background to understanding circadian rhythms in human performance, the rhythms of relevant physiological systems at rest are briefly described in this chapter.

2.2 Body temperature

The body temperature shows a distinct cyclic variation throughout the solar day. It is often used as a marker rhythm because of its ease of measurement and large endogenous component (Fig. 2.1). There are other rhythms which can be attributed directly to changes in body temperature. The temperature of biological tissues affects their metabolic rate according to the Q_{10} value. For example, a Q_{10} of 2, means that the rate of metabolism is doubled for every 10 °C rise in temperature.

For thermoregulatory purposes, the body may be divided into a central part or core and a peripheral part or shell. The temperature of the core is relatively constant at about 37 °C: it is elevated by about 0.5 °C in females during the ovulatory phase of the menstrual cycle and its daily range of oscillation is about 0.6–1.0 °C. Core temperature is usually indicated by measurement of the tympanic, oesophageal, rectal, oral, or urine temperature. Tympanic temperature is a good indicator of body temperature in conditions in which there is a rapid exchange of heat with the environment. Oesophageal temperature is probably the most appropriate for experimental studies of circadian rhythms in thermoregulatory responses to exercise. Rectal temperature is preferable to oral temperature, while the temperature of midstream urine is adequate under resting conditions but limited by the frequency with which it can be measured.

The relative stability of core temperature is maintained despite changes in environmental conditions. The temperature of the body's shell is more variable and responsive to the ambient temperature. Normally, there is a

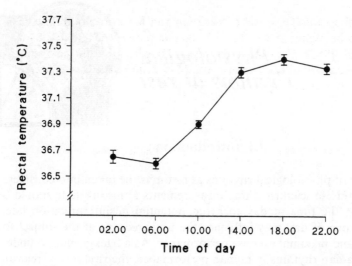

Fig. 2.1 The circadian rhythm in rectal temperature (Reilly 1994).

4 °C gradient between the core and mean skin temperatures, with a further gradient to the environment. This allows heat exchange between the organism and the environment: without a facility for losing heat to the environment, the heat gained due to metabolic processes would cause a fatal rise in core temperature within an hour. This process is accelerated during exercise when up to 80% of the energy used in muscle contractions may be dissipated as heat within the tissues.

The body temperature is regulated by clusters of cells within the hypothalamus deep within the brain. There is a heat-loss centre, which activates mechanisms for losing heat when the body temperature is rising, and a heat-gain centre, which stimulates mechanisms that protect against the cold. Increased blood flow to the skin and secretion of sweat on the skin surface promote heat loss, while heat-conserving mechanisms include vasoconstriction (to reduce skin blood flow) and elevated metabolic rate (Fig. 2.2). Clearly, the thermal state of the body represents a balance between heat-gain and heat-loss mechanisms. There is a neural link between the hypothalamic area and cells of the SCN, which, as indicated in Chapter 1, is thought to be the site of a biological clock.

Chronobiological studies of thermoregulation have entailed cooling or heating the body at different times of the day and monitoring responses. The body's thermal state can be altered rapidly by immersing, usually only part of the body, in water, or exposing the individual to a sauna or environmental chamber. In warming up after experimental cold-immersion, the blood flow to the skin is greater in the morning than in the afternoon. The peak of adrenergic activity, which would cause increased vasoconstriction and promote a rise in core temperature, occurs about midday or early in the afternoon. The threshold for onset of sweating and forearm blood flow has been reported to be higher at 16:00 and 20:00 compared to 24:00 and 04:00 (Stephenson *et al.* 1984). These observations are consistent with the conclusion that it is the *control* of body temperature rather than the loss or gain of heat that varies in a circadian cycle.

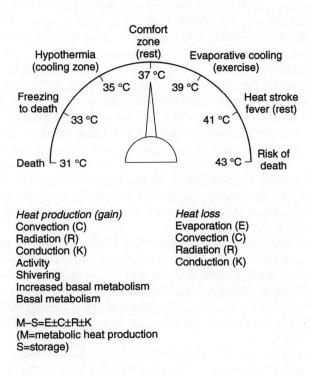

Heat production (gain)
Convection (C)
Radiation (R)
Conduction (K)
Activity
Shivering
Increased basal metabolism
Basal metabolism

Heat loss
Evaporation (E)
Convection (C)
Radiation (R)
Conduction (K)

M–S=E±C±R±K
(M=metabolic heat production
S=storage)

Fig. 2.2 Mechanisms controlling heat loss and heat gain.

2.3 Metabolism

Metabolic functions display circadian rhythmicity, independent of external factors, such as feeding, exercise, or environmental conditions. The amplitude is half the range between the peak and the trough of the rhythm. The rhythms in oxygen consumption ($\dot{V}O_2$) and in carbon dioxide production ($\dot{V}CO_2$) have an amplitude of about 7% of the mean value. This compares to a rhythm in minute ventilation ($\dot{V}E$) of about 11%. Based on calculations using a Q_{10} of 2, it has been estimated that only about one-third of the variation in metabolism can be explained by the circadian rhythm in body temperature, despite the fact that their peaks occur close to the same time of day (Reilly and Brooks 1990).

The data in Fig. 2.3 show that the curves of $\dot{V}CO_2$ and $\dot{V}O_2$ are closely in phase. This indicates that the respiratory exchange (RER) ratio ($\dot{V}CO_2/\dot{V}O_2$) does not vary with the time of day. The contribution of fats and carbohydrates to the energy produced in metabolic processes at a whole-body level is often calculated from the RER values. Measured at the cellular level, this index is referred to as the nonprotein respiratory quotient (RQ): an RQ of 0.702 would indicate the metabolism of fat while a value of 1.000 would indicate that carbohydrate is the sole source of fuel for combustion. The RER at rest is normally about 0.82. Feeding patterns during the day exert transient influences on the normally smooth circadian curve in metabolism, with a temporary elevation being known as the specific dynamic activity of food. A meal high in carbohydrates will raise the RER while a meal high in fats will decrease it slightly. There are circadian rhythms in the levels of metabolic hormones circulating in the blood. These hormones are secreted by endocrine glands, mainly in an episodic manner and varying between individuals. The separate hormonal rhythms do not fit into a classical sine-wave pattern corresponding to the smooth rhythm of $\dot{V}O_2$. This is due not just to the episodic pattern of secretion, but to the nonmetabolic functions of some of the hormones involved and their dedication to subserve specific organs and tissues.

Levels of adrenaline and noradrenaline both peak early in the afternoon and reach a nadir at night. These rhythms are more tightly linked with the sleep–wake or arousal cycle than to that of metabolism. Output from the adrenal cortex is stimulated by adrenocorticotrophic hormone (ACTH), which is secreted by the anterior pituitary gland. Serum ACTH falls at night as does serum cortisol. Each episode of cortisol secretion is preceded 10

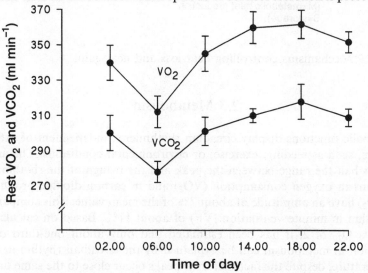

Fig. 2.3 Circadian rhythm in $\dot{V}O_2$ and $\dot{V}CO_2$ (Reilly and Brooks 1982).

min beforehand by secretion of ACTH from the pituitary. Highest cortisol levels in plasma are observed in the morning; they seem to be a function of the time at which an individual has fallen asleep but are independent of sleep itself.

Growth hormone has a metabolic function; its secretion stimulates lipid metabolism and inhibits carbohydrate metabolism. It is secreted by the anterior pituitary and has an effect throughout the body. Its levels are low during wakefulness, except for secretory bouts associated with eating or exercise. Growth hormone secretion is stimulated in response to exercise and this response is thought to have an anabolic function. Its pattern of secretion throughout the day is unrelated to plasma levels of cortisol, insulin or glucose. The elevations in GH output at night are associated with the slow-wave portion of sleep. For this reason it has been linked with restorative processes attributed to sleep by some reseachers.

Thyroid-stimulating hormone (TSH) is another anterior pituitary product which displays a circadian rhythm; it stimulates the thyroid gland to release its hormones. Thyroid hormone secretion is increased after some hours in cold ambient conditions, thus increasing heat production by means of metabolism and protecting against a fall in body temperature. However, the circadian rhythm in TSH secretion does not match the normal rhythm in $\dot{V}O_2$. Levels of TSH peak in the evening before the onset of sleep and after a decline in metabolism (as reflected by $\dot{V}O_2$). Plasma levels of TSH are elevated throughout the night and decline sharply in the morning hours to about 50% of the nighttime peak. In the absence of sleep, the evening rise is maintained nocturnally

Prolactin secretion from the pituitary reaches a peak 60–90 min after sleep onset but attains a subsequent high point about 07:00 to 08:00. During wakefulness, the levels fall to a minimum as noon approaches. Prolactin has an anabolic effect and so its rhythmic action is in concert with effects of rhythms in luteinizing hormone (LH), GH, and testosterone at a time when the catabolic effects of ACTH are lowest.

The balance of pancreatic hormones, insulin and glucagon, determines the levels of glucose in the blood and its entry into the cells. Plasma insulin levels peak during midafternoon and plasma glucagon peaks during early evening. There is a circadian variation in response to a standard glucose-tolerance test. Blood glucose and nonesterified fatty acids are elevated and the insulin response is delayed in the afternoon compared to the morning following a glucose load. A lower plasma insulin level in the morning rather than in the afternoon following a glucose load indicates that the circadian rhythm in pancreatic hormones is mainly exogenous.

2.4 Oxygen transport, blood, and circulation

The rhythm of resting minute ventilation (Fig. 2.4) is approximately sinusoidal, with values during sleep decreasing by 2 litres min^{-1} compared to the highest daytime values. There is a corresponding rightward shift of the CO_2 sensitivity curve. The vital capacity also is lower at nighttime than during the day. Changes of airway resistance are thought to be secondary to changes in the output of catecholamines from the adrenal medulla (Gaultier *et al.* 1977).

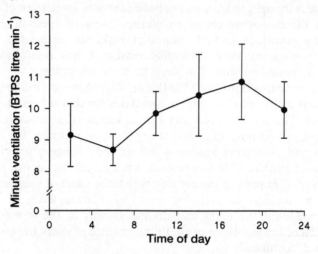

Fig. 2.4 The circadian rhythm in minute ventilation ($\dot{V}E$) (Reilly and Brooks (1982)).

The circulatory system determines the supply of oxygen throughout the body and the removal of waste products. Its effectiveness is very dependent on heart function, many parameters of which show circadian variation. The cardiac output generally peaks in the late afternoon with considerably lower values during the night (Miller and Hellander 1979). The amplitude (mean-to-peak difference) of the endogenous component of the heart-rate rhythm (Fig. 2.5) is about 4 beats min^{-1}. The total (normally observed) variation in heart rate is much greater than this due to the exogenous component. The rhythm should be taken into consideration if the pulse rate at rest is interpreted as an index of cardiovascular status as used in screening for overtraining. The rhythm in heart rate is partly determined by a timekeeper intrinsic to the heart (Tharp and Folk 1965), but is also influenced by temperature.

The time of day at which the rhythm reaches its highest point is known as the acrophase. The acrophase of the heart-rate rhythm generally occurs a few

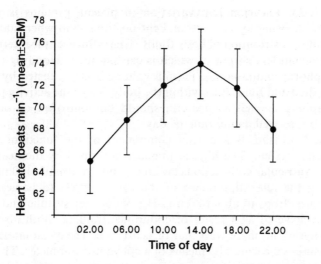

Fig. 2.5 The amplitude of the circadian rhythm in heart rate is about 4 beats min^{-1} (Reilly and Brooks 1986).

hours earlier in the day than that of the body temperature (Table 2.1). The rise in heart rate during the day includes the influence of wakefulness as well as of body temperature. This is supported by observations of cardiac function, with both the pre-ejection period and the Q-T interval of the electrocardiogram (ECG) showing circadian variation. This agrees too with the rhythms of both adrenaline and noradrenaline, which also affect the rhythms of body temperature. They also coincide with rhythms in stroke volume and blood flow to the head, which demonstrate peak values around the middle of the day or in the afternoon.

Table 2.1 Resting-rhythm in longitudinal (Reilly and Brooks 1982) and transverse (Reilly and Brooks 1990) studies.

Variable	Amplitude (% of mean)	Acrophase 24-hour clock
Heart rate	6.0–6.1	13:50–15:31
$\dot{V}E$	7.0–9.7	16:39–17:01
$\dot{V}O_2$ (litre)	6.4–6.5	17.23–17.26
$\dot{V}O_2$ (ml kg^{-1} min^{-1})	6.6–6.7	17:12–17:13
Rectal temperature	0.6–0.8	17:44–19.26

There are circadian changes also in blood composition. The rhythm in some bloodborne substances is related to meals, activity, and posture rather than to the existence of an internal clock. The changes in serum potassium, for example, are secondary to alterations in blood glucose and insulin due to intake of food. The circadian variation in plasma proteins is largely a postural effect, being lower in recumbent postures than when standing, as a result of the redistribution of body fluids. This influences the interpretation of serum calcium levels (half of which is carried in the blood by albumin), iron, phosphorus and minerals. Plasma volume is also affected by exercise, due to lost fluid and fluid shifts within the body. Thus, the activity preceding blood sampling, as well as posture, should be controlled or taken into consideration, as well as the time of day.

The blood pressure is a crucial component of the functioning of the cardiovascular system. The highest pressure generated by the heart occurs during left ventricular contractions (systole), and is normally 120 mm Hg at rest. During the relaxation-phase of the cardiac cycle (diastole), arterial blood pressure drops to about 80 mm Hg. Values for systolic and diastolic pressure are lowered as a result of endurance training. Both also show a circadian rhythm in phase with that of heart rate. The circadian rhythm in blood pressure is measured by means of a sphygmomanometer. The rhythm measured may be unreliable unless special precautions are taken, largely because blood pressure is easily distorted by external factors or by the subject's anxiety. In experimental work, an indwelling probe is employed throughout the day for continuous measurement of blood pressure to avoid such distortions. The smooth circadian rhythm in blood pressure with a peak-to-trough range of 30 mm Hg in both systolic and diastolic pressure has a different pattern in aged individuals. In the elderly, there is a subharmonic or ultradian component in the rhythm, represented by a midday peak and a rise in the afternoon following a small post-peak drop.

2.5 Renal function

Many aspects of renal function exhibit a pronounced circadian rhythm. For example, there is decreased urine output and decreased thirst intake at night. This is attributable to the pattern of pulsatile secretion of antidiuretic hormone (ADH) from the posterior pituitary gland. This hormone promotes water retention by the kidneys and its elevation during sleep reduces the requirements to void urine. The glomerular filtration rate is lowest during nighttime sleep and shows a rhythm with a 20% peak-to-trough variation. It is influenced by plasma renin activity and the hormones, angiotensin II and prostaglandins, and to a lesser extent, other hormones, such as atrial natriuretic peptide (ANP), ADH, and cortisol.

A main factor influencing renal haemodynamics (and hence renal function) is renal sympathetic nerve activity. The changes in renal function may not be so important with regard to exercise, since during exercise there is a relative shutdown of blood flow to the kidney and a redirection of blood to the active muscles. Nevertheless, monitoring the volume, timing and frequency of urine output could be useful when checking how well athletes are adapting to a new time-zone due to the shift in their circadian rhythms that this transition demands.

Circadian variations in electrolyte excretion are associated with changes in aldosterone output from the adrenal cortex. Urinary excretion of sodium, chloride, and potassium peak at about 16:00 around the time that glomerular filtration rate and renal plasma flow are highest. Aldosterone also influences blood pressure, with angiotensin. These hormones are implicated in the rhythms in systolic pressure described for the circulatory system.

The recumbent posture associated with sleep should in fact increase electrolyte excretion and urine flow. Poor kidney function is responsible for not doing so, as increased ANP prevents too much assimilation. The decrease in excretion is probably mainly due to changes in renal sympathetic activity associated with nighttime.

2.6 Nervous system

There are obviously huge changes in states of consciousness in the human between night and day. This alternation of sleep and wakefulness is matched to the dark–light cycle of the environment, which itself is linked with the spin of the earth around its long axis once every 24 hours. Not surprisingly the sleep–wake cycle is regarded as reflecting a major bodyclock, together with that directing the rhythmic changes in body temperature. There is also a rhythm in arousal and alertness, so that even during wakefulness, these in turn will influence the readiness for, and the performance of, mental, physical, and exercise tasks.

In the pineal gland, the hormone melatonin is synthesized from the compound serotonin, although there is a secondary source of melatonin within the retina. Human melatonin levels are increased at nighttime, with plasma concentrations rising from about 2 pg ml^{-1} diurnally to a nocturnal peak 30 times higher. The activity of N-acetyltransferase, an enzyme associated with the synthesis of melatonin from serotonin, also shows a pronounced rhythmic fluctuation, with nocturnal activity exceeding daytime levels by over 1000 times. Another enzyme which controls the synthesis of melatonin and whose synthesis is suppressed by light is hydroxyindole-o-methyltransferase (HIOMT). Synthesis of HIOMT is suppressed in daylight by noradrenaline released from specialized sympathetic nerve fibre relays. There are likely to be many neurotransmitter substances linked with the phenomenon of sleep, and the biological system that regulates sleep is unlikely to be explained by the concept of a single or simple 'sleep centre'. Processes associated with sleep are considered further in Chapter 5.

Noradrenaline is an important neurotransmitter in the brain: it is secreted also, as is adrenaline, by the adrenal medulla. The rhythm in noradrenaline is stronger than in adrenaline but both show a distinct circadian rhythm. This is correlated with subsequent feelings of arousal and negatively related to feelings of fatigue. In successive days without sleep, the mean values increase, demonstrating an adjustment by the body in its attempt to maintain arousal levels despite sleep deprivation. In such conditions, performance in shooting tasks has been correlated with levels of circulating catecholamines (Akerstedt *et al.* 1979).

Many performance tasks are dependent on motivational and volitional factors, and so these display greater variability than do gross motor tasks. The circadian amplitude of complex motor tasks is greater than the amplitude of those less demanding of CNS functions. It takes some time following waking before the individual is able to perform well at complex tasks. At the other extreme, there is a fatigue effect whereby performance during the day falls off due to the 'time on task'. The interactions between circadian rhythms and mental performance are covered in the next chapter (Chapter 3), and so only rhythms in basic nervous system functions are described here.

Reaction times, whether auditory or visual, tend to be fastest at the same time of day as peaks in body temperature. The same applies to sensory perception, as measured in classical vigilance tasks. Psychomotor measures, such as hand–eye coordination and pursuit motor tracking, may have a similar acrophase but peak times may occur within a broader window. Nerve-conduction velocity also displays a circadian rhythm, although its peak seems to be closer to the body-temperature curve than to that of arousal. This is compatible with findings of reduced nerve-conduction speed in cold conditions.

Mood states reflect biochemical conditions within brain cells but are typically recorded using paper-and-pencil tests. The most commonly used inventory for measuring the mood states of athletes is the mood-adjective checklist (McNair and Lorr 1964). There are circadian variations in states of vigour, activity, fatigue, inertia, and other factors, which clearly reflect the changes in arousal referred to earlier (Fig. 2.6). There is also a circadian rhythm in endogenous brain opiates; beta-endorphin levels fall at night in comparison with daytime values, although the patterns are not perfectly matched to pain tolerance.

It seems that moods associated with 'arousal' are influenced by rhythms in cortisol and catecholamines. The catecholamines lower the threshold of the reticular neurones in the brainstem, which have for many decades been linked with symptoms of drowsiness and alertness. Increased CNS levels of noradrenaline are associated with elevations in mood, particularly drive and aggression. The rhythm in cortisol is probably important in raising alertness on waking in the morning, as well as responding to stress later in the waking day.

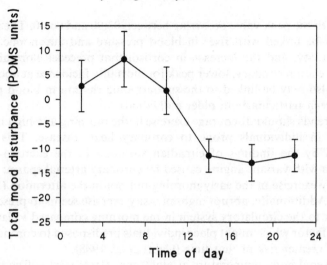

Fig. 2.6 Mood factors vary according to circadian rhythms, with peak values occurring in the afternoon and early evening.

Subjective judgements normally attributed to mental states may be influenced by both sleep–wakefulness and body-temperature rhythms. Estimation of how quickly time passes, for example, is dependent on the time of day. The usual method of time estimation is to ask subjects to count to themselves at a 1-second rate for 60 s. The rhythm in the subjective perception of time is related to a 'chemical-clock' hypothesis: the higher the body temperature, the quicker the chemical reaction, the faster the chemical clock, and the faster is the speed of counting. The chemical-clock theory is supported by observations that lower body temperature in divers leads to an underestimation of the time lapsed. It is not known whether the circadian variation in the estimation of time affects coordination tasks requiring fine timing of actions, or prolonged efforts in which motivation may decline.

2.7 Clinical implications of physical rhythms

There is a marked circadian variation in the major events of human life. The initiation of spontaneous labour prior to giving birth is most frequent after midnight and least frequent at about midday. Births occur more frequently during the night than during the day, usually about 04:00. The circadian rhythm of natural births is not replicated in the statistics for induced births which reflect the obstetric policy of inducing labour during the daytime.

There is also a prominent circadian variation in the time at which death occurs, with the peak value occurring between 03:00 and 06:00. The morning peak may be linked with rises in blood pressure and autonomic nervous system activity, and the increase in cortisol that precedes normal waking time. There is a secondary, lower peak for mortality incidence at about 16:00 and this also may be linked to the subharmonic rhythm in blood pressure, which is seen particularly in older individuals.

These trends should discourage exercise in the morning at a high intensity, especially in individuals prone to coronary heart disease. This view is supported by the findings of circadian variation in the exercise-capacity of patients with variant angina caused by coronary arterial spasm; this was induced by exercise in the early morning but not in the afternoon (Yasue *et al.* 1979). Additionally, abrupt high-intensity exercise seems to present more of a shock to the circulatory system in the morning compared to later on in the day, a factor which might place individuals predisposed to coronary heart disease at greater risk at that time (Cabri *et al.* 1988).

The lowered body temperature at nighttime affects joint stiffness, as well as functioning of soft tissues. The normal circadian rhythm in joint mobility can be altered in diseased states. Patients with rheumatoid arthritis have a normal timing of their rhythm in muscular strength, but show amplitudes three times greater than normal. Many biological rhythms are influenced by illnesses and disease, but the effects are not necessarily consistent between diseased states.

The effects that drugs have on the body are also influenced by the time at which they are administered and by the scheduling of doses. A barbiturate dose, for example, that is safe in the evening can have exaggerated effects if taken early in the morning. This has opened up a whole area of study known as chronopharmacology. It has implications for administration of medication, including the treatment of sports injuries.

2.8 Overview

There are many circadian rhythms in physiological functions evident under resting conditions, indeed most body's systems seem to exhibit circadian rhythmicity. Exercise imposes enormous perturbations on physiological systems, particularly on nervous, metabolic, circulatory, hormonal, and thermoregulatory mechanisms. The existence of circadian rhythms in exercise performance and in response to exercise merits detailed exploration. Influence of the bodyclock on exercise performance could make the difference between success and failure in a competitive contest.

Further reading

Reilly, T. (1994). Circadian rhythms. In *Oxford textbook of sports medicine* (ed. M. Harries, C. Williams, W. D. Stanish, and L. J. Micheli), pp. 238–53. Oxford University Press, New York.

Shephard, R. J. (1984). Sleep, biorhythms and human performance. *Sports Med.*, 1, 11.

Winget, C. M., D. Roshia, C. W., and Holley, D. C. (1985). Circadian rhythms and athletic performance. *Med. Sci. Sports Exerc.*, 17, 497–516.

Winget, G. M., Soliman, M. R. I., Holley, D. C., and Meyler, J. S. (1992). Chronobiology of physical performance and sports medicine. In *Biological rhythms in clinical and laboratory medicine* (ed. Y. Touitou and E. Haus), pp.229–242. Springer-Verlag, Berlin.

References

Akerstedt, T., Froberg, J. E., Friberg, Y., and Wetterberg, L. (1979). Melatonin excretion, body temperature and subjective arousal during 64 hours of sleep deprivation. *Psychoendocrinol.*, 4: 219–25.

Cabri, J., Clarys, J. P., De Witte, B., Reilly, T., and Strass, D. (1988). Circadian variation in blood pressure responses to muscular exercise. *Ergonomics*, 31, 1559–66.

Gaultier, C., Reinberg, A., and Girard, F. (1977). Circadian rhythms in lung resistance and dynamic lung compliance of healthy children. Effects of two bronchodilators. *Respir. Physiol.*, 31, 169–82.

McNair, D. M. and Lorr, M. (1964). An analysis of mood in neurotics. *J. Abnorm. Social Psychol.*, 69, 620–7.

Miller, J. C. and Hellander, M. (1979). The 24-hour cycle and nocturnal depression of cardiac output. *Aviat., Space Environ. Med.*, 50, 1139–44.

Reilly, T. and Brooks, G. A. (1982). Investigation of circadian rhythms in metabolic responses to exercise. *Ergonomics*, 25, 1093–7.

Reilly, T. and Brooks, G. A. (1990). Selective persistence of circadian rhythms in physiological responses to exercise. *Chronobiol. Int.*, 7, 59–67.

Stephenson, L. A., Winger, C. B., O'Donovan, B. H., and Nadel, E. R. (1984). Circadian rhythms in sweating and cutaneous blood flow. *Amer. J. Physiol.*, 246, R321–R324.

Tharp, G. D. and Folk, Jr., G. E. (1965). Rhythmic changes in data of mammalian heart and heart cells during prolonged isolation. *Comparat. Physiol. Biochem*, 14, 255–73.

Yasue, H., Omote, S., Takizawa, A., Naguo, M., Miwa, K., and Tanaka, S. (1979). Circadian variation of exercise capacity in patients with Prinzmetal's variant angina: role of exercise-induced coronary arterial spasm. *Circulation*, 59, 938.

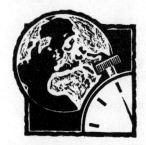

3

Circadian rhythms in mental performance

A successful athlete needs to be at the peak of his or her mental capacities when competing. Do mental processes show circadian rhythmicity? If so, when are the best times for skills requiring vigilance, decision-taking and precision movements? It is these issues that will be the topics of this chapter.

3.1 Measuring mental performance during the normal day

There has been no systematic research which specifically deals with chronobiological aspects of mental performance in athletes. The majority of work has been done, both in the laboratory and in field studies, upon healthy volunteers, often in a shiftworking context.

3.1.1 Standardizing tests of mental performance

Measuring performance in field studies is beset by problems. First, many work-tasks are difficult to quantify. This is the case if the task involves decision-taking, for which a quantitative assessment can seldom be made, or if there is no end-product that can be examined (e.g. teaching or watch-keeping on night-duty). Even if a task can be assessed quantitatively, a further difficulty may arise from a lack of standardization of the task itself. For example, different demands are placed on the workforce, according to whether the work is paced by the individual or by some external influence (e.g. the speed at which a conveyor-belt moves). In addition, the conditions, where the task is being carried out often vary considerably (e.g. driving a vehicle or working outdoors), or they differ from one worksite to another (e.g. lighting, noise), so that making comparisons between studies is very difficult. Finally, the physiological state of the workforce – how much sleep loss it suffers from, or how long is the duty period – can rarely be controlled. Nevertheless, those studies that have been accomplished in the field (Folkard 1990; Hildebrandt *et al.* 1974), show that accidents and errors due to human failing are more likely to occur at night. Such findings suggest that a circadian rhythm of mental performance, with a trough at night, is a contributory factor.

Many of the difficulties of interpretation associated with field studies can be controlled or the differences quantified (and hence corrected for statistically) in a laboratory environment. Subjects' conditions of work and, to some extent, their lifestyles, can also be controlled more closely, as well as the detailed nature of the tasks they perform.

For studies directly applicable to athletes, the same general problems apply. Thus, there has rarely been a standardization of environmental conditions or of the type of athletic task or individual, as would be required in order to compare results. Even in the laboratory, there is a need to standardize exercise tests in simulations of sport performance.

The earlier tasks used in laboratory experiments tended to be pencil-and-paper tests. More recently, tests have become more automated, with test answers being recorded on portable tape-recorders or personal computers, with the questions also being asked by these devices. There is the added advantage that the answers can be scored automatically.

A plethora of tasks has been used by researchers. Nevertheless, they can be classified into the following main types: subjective assessments, simple objective tests, and more complex objective assessments (Folkard and Monk, 1985; Minors and Waterhouse 1981).

3.1.1.1 Subjective assessments

These measure mood, often by requiring the subject to mark a line somewhere between its ends, which indicate 'not at all' or 'as much as possible' to a question like 'How alert do you feel?'

3.1.1.2 Simple objective assessments

There are very many of these but they tend to focus upon some aspect of sensory, cognitive or manipulative ability, upon short-term memory, or upon some combination of these. Visual-search tasks would constitute a test dominated by the speed and accuracy of perception of sensory input. Manipulative skill might be assessed by, for example, threading beads onto a string, or inserting ball-bearings of slightly different sizes into holes of the appropriate size. Logical reasoning can be assessed by sets of syllogisms or by a logical reasoning test in which a pair of letters 'A, B' are presented as either 'A, B' or 'B, A' and the subject is asked to say whether a statement such as 'B is not followed by A' is true or false.

Short-term memory has been assessed by means of a search-and-memory test (Folkard *et al.* 1976). A block of random letters is given and each line has to be scanned separately for a 'target' of between two and six letters. As the length of the target increases, so does the extent to which short-term memory, in addition to visual search, is required to accomplish the task.

Reaction-time has been measured in several ways. Simple reaction-time is the delay between receiving a signal (visual or auditory) and responding to it, generally by pressing a button. The task can be made more complex by requiring the subject, in choice reaction-time, to respond to a stimulus with the correct choice of response – for example, extinguishing the correct light from a choice of four when it becomes illuminated. These tests of reaction-time can be changed also by altering the amount of warning given to the subject before the stimulus is given.

3.1.1.3 More complex assessments – the problem of 'realism'

The above tasks enable the mood and several aspects of mental performance to be assessed under circumstances that are standardized and better controlled – and so more scientifically reliable than real tasks. But the element of 'realism' has been sacrificed; real tasks are often a combination of the above, and much more complex.

There are several ways in which complexity can be added to tests, such as those described above. First, the task itself can be made more difficult, involving more thought or a combination of skills. Examples of the former are mental addition or plotting Cartesian coordinates, while examples of the latter include tracking a moving object, copying meaningless symbols, and substituting digits for symbols. The use of video-games has been suggested, with separate scores being kept of the various types of skill demanded by the games (Kennedy *et al.* 1982). Another possibility is to mix together a battery of tasks, the components of which can remain simple (Alluisi 1972). The overall workload can be increased by putting time constraints on the subjects, particularly if they are required to act upon, or choose, priorities when several tasks are presented simultaneously. This introduces the concept of 'workload', too much of which can give rise to 'stress'. Indeed, tests to produce just such a reaction in the subject have been designed (e.g. Patkai 1971). It is a small step only from these complexities to the use of flight-simulators, but this last possibility takes us almost full circle. Thus, while flight-simulation is more 'real' than the other tasks described above, its sheer complexity poses problems if the different factors involved in performance need to be separated out. The equipment needed would also be costly to run and unsuited to carrying from one site to another.

Vigilance is one aspect of 'realism' that can be duplicated in the laboratory. Vigilance requires the individual to recognize and respond to an event that occurs infrequently. It can be assessed by inserting abnormal stimuli – or missing them out altogether – into repetitive stimuli that form a 'normal' background. The stimuli can be auditory or visual, and realism can be added by including additional tasks that tend to distract the attention (see above). Tasks requiring vigilance are different from most others in that they require much longer to perform – hours rather than minutes.

3.2 Circadian rhythms in performance

Figure 3.1 shows some rhythms of alertness and performance that have been measured throughout the waking hours in healthy subjects living a conventional sleep–activity schedule. Clearly, there are rhythmic changes, with lowest values in the early morning and late evening for most variables. Not unexpectedly, the values are also lower when measurements are made after waking up subjects during the night. Thus, during the night, there are negative and unfavourable effects upon mental state and performance in several types of mental task.

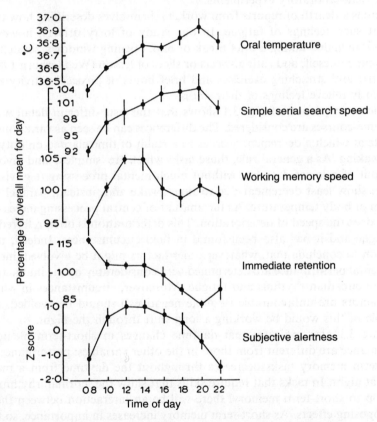

Fig. 3.1 Time-course of oral temperature, some types of mental performance, and subjective alertness during the daytime in healthy subjects (Folkard 1990). The use of a Z score for alertness is explained on p. 148.

Poorer performance and lower arousal at night – associated with an increased degree of sleepiness – are bad enough, but they can be associated with worse difficulties, particularly in field conditions. First, individuals can suffer from becoming drowsy or even show overt sleep episodes. Second, a rather unusual phenomenon called nightshift paralysis can occur, in which individuals, though apparently awake, nevertheless become immobile and are unable to respond to their environment. It lasts from a few seconds to minutes and has been described in nurses and airtraffic controllers (Folkard and Condon 1987). These phenomena do not seem to have been observed in laboratory studies, though extremely long delays in tests of reaction-time or missed signals in vigilance tests (see below) have both been found and might have some affinity. This failure to duplicate field results exactly acts as a reminder, however, that real tasks are supervized far less and last so much longer than laboratory experiments.

There is a dearth of reports from workers themselves describing how they combat such feelings of fatigue. In one study of lorry drivers, however, methods included taking a brief break or nap, opening windows, scratching or slapping oneself, and eating sweets or slices of lemon (Wedderburn 1987). Isometric and stretching exercises and brief bouts of physical activity also transiently relieve feelings of drowsiness.

A closer inspection of Fig. 3.1 shows that the tests differ in detail when their time-courses are considered. The differences can be seen as variations in the rate at which a decrement accrues as a result of time elapsed on duty or since waking. As a general rule, those tasks which are 'simplest' and involve the input of a lot of data but without much mental processing (e.g. visual search) show least decrement due to time awake and, instead, parallel the rhythm of body temperature. As the amount of central processing increases, so too does the speed of deterioration. This deterioration is often referred to as fatigue and it has also been found in field circumstances. Indeed, it is common to conclude that, whatever other factors might be involved, mood and mental performance are determined very considerably by the interaction between circadian rhythms and fatigue. Moreover, circumstances in which both factors are unfavourable ('double negatives') should be avoided. An example of this would be working a long shift through the night.

Figure 3.1 also indicates that daytime changes in short-term memory performance are different from those in the other variables: performance at short-term memory tasks decreases throughout the daytime from a maximum at night. In tasks that require skills that show the 'normal' rhythm in addition to short-term memory, there will be an interaction between these two opposing effects. As short-term memory increases in importance, so the peak of the rhythm shifts from the late daytime towards nighttime.

3.3 Vigilance, workload, and motivation

Like many other mental tasks, vigilance shows circadian changes, with minimum vigilance at night, and deteriorates with time spent on the task.

Nevertheless, it is clear that vigilance is affected also by several other factors, among which are motivation and workload.

Highly motivated individuals wish to perform at their peak. As we have seen, this peak might be lower at night, but it is affected also by sleep loss (Section 3.5) and the task itself. Interest promotes performance, and ways to increase interest are important. One method is to give the individual feedback about performance; for athletes, this amounts to training in such a way that a good performance can be aimed for and realized as such while it is being achieved. Another way to maintain motivation is to change the task as often as reasonable, thereby reducing monotony to which, of course, vigilance is especially prey. Interest can be maintained also by having enough, but not too many, errors to deal with. If there are too few, the individual gets bored, while if there are too many, the individual becomes overwhelmed. This takes us to the concept of workload.

Evaluating workload has been attempted in several ways. First, the severity of the task itself can sometimes be assessed objectively as, for example, the number of aircraft dealt with per hour by an airtraffic controller. Second, the assessment can be more subjective, originating from the workforce itself or from independent observers. Third, physiological changes associated with mental effort can be measured. (The difference between 'alert' and 'stressed' seems rather arbitrary here). Possible variables are heart rate and its variability, blood pressure, body temperature, and plasma or urinary catecholamines.

Correlations between these variables and other estimates of workload can be high and positive, but this close matching is not invariably the case. The lack of a high correlation between the stimulus and subjective or objective responses to it might provide us with some understanding of the problem. Thus, if the workload increases, so too should the individual's responses. If the response is too high – 'stressed' seems a useful concept here – or if it is too low (through overconfidence, lack of attention, or boredom), then accidents and errors become more likely. In order to perform at peak efficiency, an individual needs to achieve a balance between effort and workload.

3.4 Ultradian components of mental performance

In addition to circadian rhythms of performance, ultradian rhythms exist also. The best known is the temporary decline in performance in the early afternoon – the 'post-lunch dip'. There is controversy about whether the dip is caused by having eaten lunch and whether or not other circadian rhythms (e.g. adrenaline, body temperature) are affected. Recent work suggests that a decrement does occur, in some people and in some performance tasks, that is related to having eaten a meal. This decline is not invariably reflected in a fall of body temperature (the significance of this is discussed in Section 3.6).

3.5 Fatigue and sleep loss

Performance deteriorates with the amount of time spent on a task, particularly if vigilance is required, and can be viewed as a type of fatigue. A loss of sleep may also lead to fatigue, as might occur in the days after a time-zone transition (Chapter 6). The most common way to study loss of sleep has been to consider the effects of complete, or almost complete loss of sleep, for three or more days. There are also some studies where the effects of more modest (and common) sleep losses have been investigated.

One group of studies has been performed upon medical staff. Poulton *et al.* (1978) found that performance in a logical reasoning test fell if the subject had worked for more than 18 hours or had lost more than 3 hours of sleep. In addition, a series of haematology reports was concocted for assessment, one quarter of which had grossly abnormal results. Sleep deficits led to a more variable rate of working rather than to an increase in errors when assessing these reports. This result was attributed to the process of 'compensation'. This is one in which extra effort is required by the individual to achieve an acceptable level of performance (judged by the individual concerned), in spite of the negative factors present. A similar conclusion – that the effects of a limited degree of sleep loss could be compensated for – was reached in another study on doctors which measured several mood and mental tests (Orton and Gruzelier 1989).

Laboratory-based tests and other field studies upon shiftworkers have yielded similar, if not identical, results. That is, circadian rhythms continue, but peaks of mood and performance, and especially mood and performance in the middle of the night, all tend to fall with increasing sleep loss. These effects are more marked if the task is complex or demands vigilance, but rather less marked if the tasks require less decision-taking, such as visual search. A decreased speed of performance and an increase in erratic performance are also common findings. Clearly, maintaining reliable performance levels for extended periods of time is likely to be compromised.

3.5.1 The role of naps

The effects of sleep loss may be ameliorated by taking a nap (Naitoh 1981). Its benefits depend on the time of day it is taken, the kind of performance engaged in, the time on the task, and so on (Stampi *et al.* 1990). Naps can also offset the effects of fatigue and in particular refresh athletes for training and competing in the evening. On the downside, there is the phenomenon of sleep inertia; this is the short-term decrease in alertness experienced upon waking up (Dinges 1992). These are discussed in more detail in Chapter 5.

3.6 The origin of rhythms of mental performance

The parallelism between simple repetitive tasks (e.g. visual search) and body temperature has been mentioned already. Does this parallelism indicate a causal link? Certainly, it is conceivable that a raised temperature would promote the biochemical reactions occurring in the brain, but what evidence is there to support the causal hypothesis?

It has been argued that there is not a causal link, basing the case on the failure to find a significant positive correlation between body temperature and mental-performance score at that time, particularly during nightwork. Also, the effects of raising or lowering body temperature – to produce predictable changes in mental performance – are complex to interpret due to other influences. Thus, for example, producing a low-grade fever in individuals or cooling them by immersion in cold water are both likely to change the subjects' motivation or even produce some degree of stress! However, Åkerstedt and Folkard (1995) and Minors *et al.* (1986), by measuring alertness and mental performance in subjects on abnormal sleep–activity schedules, have been able to separate changes in these variables into two components. One component is a function of the amount of time that has elapsed since sleep and would appear to include an effect due to waking up and another due to fatigue; the other component is sinusoidal and in phase with the rhythm of body temperature. Even though such results are not proof of a causal link between mental activity and temperature, they do suggest that a parallelism exists. In addition, a similar conclusion – of a general parallelism – can be drawn when the time-courses of plasma catecholamines and mental-performance tests are considered.

Considering body temperature, catecholamine levels, and mental performance together, the concept arises of 'arousal' being a link between them all. This can then be incorporated quite readily into another concept, namely the 'inverted U' relationship between arousal and mental performance. Performance improves with increasing arousal up to an optimal point, beyond which performance levels fall with further increases in arousal. Adapting this concept to the current argument, *arousal* is produced by wide areas of the CNS. It shows circadian changes and manifests itself not only in effects upon mental performance, but also upon rhythms of body temperature and catecholamine release into the blood. Arousal is decreased by fatigue and lack of sleep and raised by activity. Sleep loss will therefore, affect performance adversely and excessive arousal – due to stress and/or mental overloading – will push the individual past the peak of the 'inverted U' curve, again decreasing effective performance.

Tasks with a high short-term memory component show inverse circadian rhythms. Does this indicate that this task is controlled by a separate oscillator? – Quite possibly. In addition, the rhythm of short-term memory separates from other mental-performance rhythms. For example, it dissociates from the temperature rhythm on non-24-hour 'days'. Normally, this would be regarded as a strong argument for the presence of more than one oscillator, but mental performance data are necessarily collected only during waking hours, and the effect of this upon estimates of timing and period can be difficult to determine precisely. At the moment, therefore, the explanation of the rhythm in short-term memory remains to be found.

3.7 Overview

Mood and mental performance are influenced by three main factors: rhythmicity, the quantity of recent sleep, and the amount of time spent awake. For the athlete, there are therefore clearly times of the day and circumstances (sleep loss) when those aspects of their training and competitive performance involving mental performance and motivation will feel and be less good.

Such circumstances may arise if events interfere with their daily routine, but they may be particularly marked after a change in habits, such as occurs during nightwork or after a time-zone transition. These will be discussed in detail in Chapters 6 and 8.

Further reading

Wilkinson, R. T. (1972). Sleep deprivation – eight questions. In *Aspects of human efficiency* (ed. W. P. Colquhoun). pp.25–30. English Universities Press, London.

References

Åkerstedt, T. and Folkard, S. (1995). Validation of the S and C components of the three-process model of alertness regulation. *Sleep*, 18, 1–6.

Alluisi, E. (1972). Influence of work–rest scheduling and sleep loss on sustained performance. In *Aspects of human efficiency* (ed. W. P. Colquhoun). pp.199–215. English Universities Press, London.

Dinges, D. (1992). Adult napping and its effect on ability to function. In *Why we nap* (ed. C. Stampi), pp.118–34. Birkhauser, Boston.

Folkard, S. (1990). Circadian performance rhythms: some practical and theoretical implications. *Phil. Trans. Roy. Soc., London*, Series B, 327, 543–53.

Folkard, S. and Condon, R. (1987). Night-shift paralysis in air traffic control officers. *Ergonomics*, 30, 1353–63.

Folkard, S. and Monk, T. H. (1985). Circadian performance rhythms. In *Hours of work* (ed S. Folkard and T. H. Monk), pp.37–52. Wiley, Chichester.

Folkard, S., Monk, T., and Knauth, P. (1976). The effect of memory load on the circadian variation in performance efficiency under a rapidly rotating shift system. *Ergonomics*, 19, 479–88.

Hildebrandt, G., Rohmert, W., and Rutenfranz, R. (1974). 12 and 24 h rhythms in error frequency of locomotive drivers. *Int. J. Chronobiol.*, **2**, 175–80.

Kennedy, R., Bittner, A., Harbeson, M., and Jones, B. (1982). Television computer games: a new look in performance testing. *Aviat. Space Environ. Med.*, **53**, 49–53.

Minors, D. and Waterhouse, J. (1981). *Circadian rhythms and the human*. Wright, Bristol.

Minors, D. and Waterhouse, J. (1986). Circadian rhythms and their mechanisms. *Experientia*, **42**, 1–13.

Naitoh, P. (1981). Circadian cycles and the restorative power of naps. In *Biological rhythms, sleep and shift work* (ed. L. Johnson, D. Tepas, W. Colquhoun, and M. Colligan), pp.553–80. Spectrum, New York.

Orton, D. and Gruzelier, J. (1989). Adverse changes in mood and cognitive performance of house officers after night duty. *Brit. Med. J.*, **298**, 21–3.

Patkai, P. (1971). Interindividual differences in diurnal variations in alertness, performance and adrenaline excretion. *Acta Physiol. Scand.* **81**, 35–46.

Poulton, E., Hunt, G., Carpenter, A., and Edwards, R. (1978). The performance of junior hospital doctors following reduced sleep and long hours of work. *Ergonomics*, **21**, 279–95.

Stampi, C., Broughton, R., Mullington, J., Rivers M., and Campos J. (1990). Ultrashort sleep strategies during sustained operations: the recuperative value of multiple 80-, 50- and 20-min naps. In Shiftwork: *health, sleep and performance* (ed. G. Costa, G. Cesana, K. Kogi, and A. Wedderburn). Peter Lang, Frankfurt.

Wedderburn, A. (1987). Sleeping on the job: the use of anecdotes for recording rare but serious events. *Ergonomics*, **30**, 1229–33.

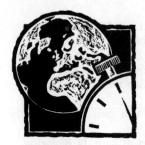

4
Circadian rhythms in sports performance

4.1 Introduction

The majority of the resting physiological variables mentioned in Chapter 2 are thought to influence human performance. For example, when body temperature, circulating levels of hormones and metabolic functions are manipulated artificially prior to exercise (e.g. by prewarming subjects or by pharmacological agents), performance is affected. Endogenous circadian changes in these resting parameters might mediate parallel changes in both performance and physiological responses to exercise over a 24-hour period. In this chapter, the evidence for such rhythmicity in human physical performance is analysed.

The chronobiology of sport and exercise has been researched in three ways which can be ordered in terms of scientific validity. First, the times of day when athletes perform the best (or worst) in actual sports events have been examined. Second, performances in simulated competitions or time-trials have been investigated at different times of the day. Finally, the responses to recognized laboratory tests of performance have been examined in rigorously controlled environments.

4.2 Indirect evidence of circadian variation in performance

World records in sports events are usually broken by athletes competing in the early evening, which is the time of day at which body temperature is highest. The mid-eighties series of middle-distance records broken by the British runners, Sebastian Coe, Steve Cram, Steve Ovett, and Dave Moorcroft, illustrates this perfectly, since all were set between 19:00 and 23:00. Such observations should of course be interpreted with caution, since there is a bias towards scheduling the finals of track and field competitions in the afternoon whereas world record attempts are associated with evening meetings due to extraneous influences, such as peak television-viewing time and the availability of spectators. In some sports, the bias towards scheduling events for the early evening can be controlled for. In the discipline of competitive cycling known as time-trialling, the frequency of races is more evenly distributed throughout the daylight hours. The performances of young competitors in 16 km races are better when held in the afternoon and evening compared to those scheduled in the morning (Atkinson *et al.* 1994*a*). When the frequency of trials is standardized at different times of day in simulated competitions, weight-throwers also perform better in the evening than in the morning (Reilly 1990).

The lack of control over environmental influences on performance is the major problem with this evidence from field studies. For instance, environmental temperature may be more favourable to record-breaking performances in the evening, especially in summer. Circadian fluctuations in meteorological conditions, such as wind speed and direction, may also affect performances in cycling or field sports involving high velocities of projectiles (e.g. discus, javelin, hammer). Nevertheless, tighter control can be exerted in swimming, as water conditions can be held constant. When this is done, the best times for 100-metre and 400-metre swims occur, again, in late afternoon or early evening (Fig. 4.1).

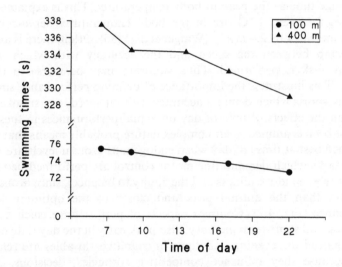

Fig. 4.1 The effects of time of day on 100-metre and 400-metre swimming time-trials (Baxter and Reilly, 1983).

4.3 Components of performance measured in the laboratory

In order to remove the above influences, experiments have been performed which control for their effects. The research design employed in these studies is described in Chapter 11.

'Performance' is a very broad term and sports events usually comprise a cocktail of task components. The predominant component of performance may vary enormously from one athletic event to another. For example, the requirements of marathon running (the ability to sustain prolonged submaximal exercise) are completely different from those of 100-metre sprinting (fast reaction-time, high short-term power output). Some events bring together a whole range of performance components which may have different circadian characteristics. For example, it is shown below that hand-steadiness peaks in the morning, whereas isometric grip-strength is highest in the afternoon or early evening. Both these components are required in a sport such as archery. In this section, an attempt is made to isolate each component of sports performance and describe the circadian characteristics of each.

4.3.1 Rhythms in psychomotor performance and motor skills

Simple reaction-time (either to auditory or visual stimuli) is a major component of performances in sprint events. It peaks in the early evening at the same time as the peak in body temperature . This is explained by the fact that, for every 1 °C rise in the body temperature, nerve-conduction veolcity increases by 2.4 m s^{-1} (Winget *et al.* 1985). Often, there is an inverse relationship between the speed and the accuracy with which a simple repetitive task is performed. Thus, accuracy may be worse in the early evening. This illustrates the importance of defining performance since there are many sports which demand accuracy without speed, e.g. snooker, darts. Although the effects of time of day on actual performances in these sports have not been examined, their complex nature probably means that they are performed best at times of day when endogenous arousal levels are lowered. Similar tasks which demand fine motor control are performed better in the morning (e.g. hand-steadiness and the ability to balance), since arousal levels are lower than the diurnal peak and closer to the optimum level for performance (Fig. 4.2). Complex aspects of performance, such as mental arithmetic and short-term memory, also peak early in the day (late morning) rather than in the evening. Rhythms in cognitive variables are relevant to sport because they influence competitive strategies, decisions, and the delivery and recall of complex coaching instructions.

Mood states and subjective alertness may be important for human performance since they may alter an individual's predisposition for strenuous physical efforts. Alertness and positive mood states peak in the waking hours (usually in the evening). Conversely, sleepiness and fatigue peak in the early hours of the morning. Mental readiness for extreme efforts is essential to the realization of performance capabilities. Circadian variations in mood states may also affect the 'team cohesion' of a work-group. For example, the ability to communicate and work together as a team is important for the effective functioning of aircraft flightdeck personnel.

The ability to estimate time also varies with the time of day. In the afternoon when body temperature is high, time intervals are overestimated

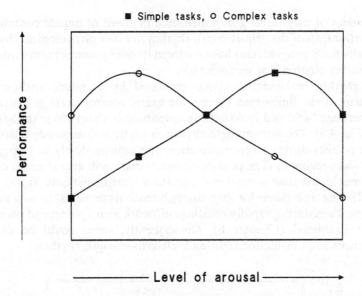

Fig. 4.2 The 'inverted U' relationship between levels of arousal and performance. The optimum level of arousal is lower for complex tasks compared to simple tasks.

(a 30-second time period presented to people would be perceived as, say, 33 s). This agrees with the 'chemical-clock' hypothesis whereby biochemical processes related to the perception of time are accelerated by raised levels of body temperature. It remains unclear whether such a phenomenon influences an athlete's subjective evaluation of 'speed' during training sessions performed at different times of the day.

Circadian rhythms in psychomotor performance, particularly tasks that entail cognitive operations seem especially prone to a 'post-lunch dip'. This phenomenon describes a transient decline in alertness and performance occurring early in the afternoon. Some aspects of performance deteriorate at this time without a corresponding decrease in body temperature and even if no food is ingested at lunchtime. This time of day should be avoided when the coach is trying to impart new skills or tactics to a group of athletes.

4.3.2 Muscle strength

A much explored variable in chronobiology, mainly because of its ease of measurement, is hand-grip strength. This variable, although moderately correlated with lean body mass and whole-body strength, is limited in the context of sport, considering the specificity of strength in different sports. Despite this, muscle strength consistently peaks in the early evening, independent of the muscle group measured or speed of muscle contraction. The relationship of the grip-strength rhythm to other physiological rhythms (especially body temperature) has promoted its use by some chronobiologists as a 'marker rhythm' for performance.

The rhythm in isometric (force generated by a muscle without any movement of the limbs that the muscle exerts control over) grip-strength peaks between 14:00 and 19:00 with an amplitude of about 6% of the 24-hour mean (Fig. 4.3). The grip-strength rhythm is partly endogenously controlled since it persists during sleep deprivation and adjusts slowly to changes in sleep – wake regimens. The peak-to-trough variation in grip strength can be three times higher than normal in rheumatoid arthritic patients (Harkness *et al.* 1982). The time taken for grip-strength rhythms to adjust to new sleep – wake schedules during rapidly rotating shiftwork seems to depend on which hand is examined (Chapter 8). Consequently, there could be distinct mechanisms responsible for right and left grip-strength rhythms.

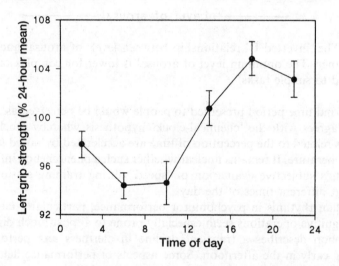

Fig. 4.3 The circadian rhythm in left-grip strength. (Unpublished data obtained from 20 subjects in the laboratory at Liverpool John Moores University).

Two diurnal peaks are found when the isometric strength of the knee extensors is measured consecutively during the waking hours of the solar day; one peak occurs at the end of the morning and the other in the late afternoon or early evening (Reilly 1990). Performance transiently declines between these times of day. Similarly, there can be a drop in grip strength between 13:00 and 14:00 when the variable is measured every hour for a 24-hour period. It is difficult to separate a true time-of-day effect from influences resulting from the experimental protocol comprising serial texts. This afternoon decline in performance may be due to the fall in motivation arising from the many consecutive (uncounter balanced) measurements taken. Despite this, when isometric strength measures are recorded under the optimal experimental protocol outlined in Chapter 11 (which allows sufficient recovery between test sessions without disturbing sleep), post-lunch declines in performance still occur (Fig. 4.4*a*). With respect to the isometric strength of other muscle groups, elbow-flexion strength varies with the time of day, peaking in the early evening (mean to peak difference). Back strength is also higher in the evening than in the morning, with an amplitude of about 6% of the 24-hour mean (Coldwells *et al.* 1993*a*).

Both concentric (generation of force while the muscle is shortening) and eccentric (generation of force while the muscle is lengthening) strength have been measured at different times of the solar day using isokinetic dynamometry (e.g. Cybex or Lido equipment). A time-of-day effect in these variables has been noted with peak values occurring in the early evening, though this is apparent only when measured at slow $(1.05–3.14$ rad s$^{-2})$ angular velocities of movement (Fig. 4.4*b*). The coefficient of variation of measurements made with computer-controlled dynamometers may be as high as 20% at fast angular velocities $(>6$ rad s$^{-1})$. Unless this error is reduced through multiple trials, it is probably too large to detect any circadian variation. Inadequate sensitivity of measuring equipment is a problem in chronobiological research and may explain why rhythms have not been detected in some other performance variables.

The maximal force generated in a test of muscle strength is referred to as a maximal voluntary contraction. This is dependent on central (motivation) and peripheral (neuromuscular) factors. It is still not known which of these factors predominates in the circadian rhythm in muscular strength.

4.3.3 Short-term power output

When pretest protocols are identical, it is difficult to detect circadian rhythms in computer-interfaced tests of anaerobic power such as the 'Wingate test' (a 30-second all-out test on a cycle ergometer during which work-rate is recorded every second). This is true for both leg and arm ergometry. Vigorous warm-up procedures prior to administration of the tests may 'swamp' any rhythm that may be present. In addition, the sensitivity of the ergometry used in the Wingate test may be insufficient to detect such small amplitude rhythms.

Simpler criteria of performance, such as the duration that a set high-intensity work-rate can be maintained, do vary with the time of day. Longer worktimes and higher peaks of lactate production occur when set high-intensity exercise is performed in the evening (22:00) compared to morning

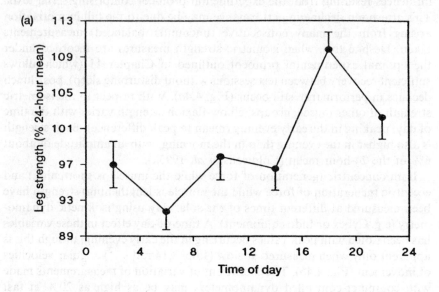

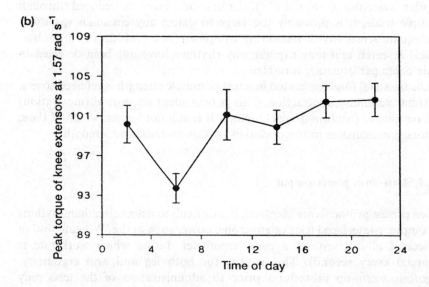

Fig. 4.4 Circadian rhythms in leg strength: (a) isometric strength of the knee extensors measured with a spring-loaded dynamometer; (b) isokinetic strength of the knee extensors measured at an angular velocity of 1.57 rad s^{-1}. (Unpublished data obtained from 20 subjects in the laboratory at Liverpool John Moores University).

(06:30) (Reilly 1990). The time of day also influences the performance of all-out explosive efforts. Performance in the standing broad-jump shows a circadian rhythm with an acrophase of 17:45 and an amplitude of about 3% of the 24-hour mean (Reilly and Down 1986). Similar rhythm characteristics are found for vertical-jumping performance. Since the performances of medal winners in jumping events are often within a few centimetres of each other, the time of day should therefore be recognized as a significant factor in such events. It is particularly relevant when an athlete has to meet certain performance standards to qualify for major championships.

The evening superiority of swim performances measured 'in the pool' is likely to be physiological in origin, since mean and peak power outputs recorded on a swim bench under controlled conditions still vary with time of day. Amplitudes of these rhythms are 11–14% of 24-hour mean values and the acrophase is about 18:00 (Reilly and Marshall 1991). These amplitudes are greater than those found for muscular strength, possibly due to the more complex motor coordination required of the upper limbs in simulated swimming.

4.4 Physiological responses to exercise

Presuming that the magnitude of the masking effect of exercise on circadian rhythms does not vary with time of day, it might be deduced that physiological rhythms in resting variables would be maintained during exercise. Some rhythms, however, disappear, whereas others become more marked during exercise. This could be attributable to experimental errors, such as a failure to control prior activity and diet of the subjects, or to the increases in arousal which may precede exercise. The intensity of exercise and fitness of the subjects may also influence exercise circadian rhythms. For example, the fluctuations might be too small for detection in responses to high-intensity exercise. Despite these effects, several conclusions can be drawn from the evidence that is currently available.

4.4.1 Body temperature

Since fluctuations in body temperature are believed to mediate many circadian rhythms in performance, the characteristics of this rhythm during exercise are important. The acrophase and amplitude of the rhythm in rectal temperature remain unchanged during exercise (Reilly and Brooks 1986). Rhythms in skin temperature during exercise are generally in phase with their corresponding resting rhythms but depend on the site of measurement. For instance, skin temperature of the limbs used in cycle ergometry does not seem to vary with the time of day due to the cooling effect of the limb movements themselves.

During endurance races in the heat, athletes may have to exercise with their body temperatures above the level conducive to optimal performance and close to temperatures normally indicative of heat injury. Thus, if endurance exercise is carried out in the evening, there is an increased likelihood that such body temperatures will be attained, since as stated above, the body temperature rhythm is maintained during exercise (Reilly 1990). Although a set body-temperature threshold for heat injury has yet to be confirmed, assuming that a threshold is constant throughout the day, the margin of safety for heat injury can be calculated to be 0.5 °C greater in the morning than in the afternoon.

Evidence from two sources supports the assertion that, in fit subjects, performance in sustained exercise is influenced by a lower body temperature similar to that found in the morning. First, if the body temperature is precooled, prior to 1 hour exercise, by an amount that corresponds to the amplitude of the circadian rhythm, this will cause a significant increase in work-rate (Hessemer *et al.* 1984). Inferences from this to circadian variation must, however, be made with caution because of the different factors altering the body-temperature setpoint. Second, there is a significant interaction between the work-rate, measured every 10 min during 80 min of submaximal exercise, and the time of day (Atkinson *et al.* 1994c). In the evening, when body temperature is highest, subjects choose greater work-rates at the beginning of the exercise period in the evening compared to in the morning. However, as the body temperature rises above optimal levels during the evening exercise, so the work-rate drops. In the morning, the work-rate gradually increases as body temperature rises towards optimal levels, until, at the end of the exercise period, subjects choose higher work-rates in the morning than in the afternoon (Fig. 4.5). In cold and wet conditions, however, athletes running at very low exercise intensities (e.g. charity runners in marathon races) may be at greater risk of hypothermia in the morning. Their low work-rate may be insufficient to maintain heat balance due to the high loss of heat to the cold environment. In such conditions, appropriate clothing is needed to safeguard against a dangerous drop in the body's core temperature.

In the past, it was recognized that environmental temperature is more favourable for athletes in marathon races in the early morning. Consequently, in hot and humid conditions such as in Hong Kong, Singapore and Penang, marathons have started at 05:00–06:00. Recently, marathons have been scheduled at later times of the day to coincide with the demands of television audiences. Such scheduling may be disastrous to athletes if the environmental temperature is high. The Olympic marathon in Sydney in the year 2000 would pose a particular problem if West European and North American television companies exert their influence over the time of day that the races are held, as they did for the scheduling of matches in the 1994 soccer World Cup.

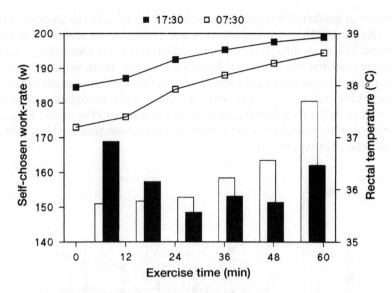

Fig. 4.5 Effects of time of day on self-chosen work-rate (bars) and rectal temperature (square numbers) during 80 min of exercise on a cycle ergometer (Atkinson *et al.* 1994*b*).

4.4.2 Cardiovascular variables

Heart rates during exercise are consistently lower at night, irrespective of work-rate, with the day–night difference amounting to 5–10 beats min^{-1} kcal's min^{-1}. This temporal pattern is also apparent in recovery heart rates following a set exercise regimen (e.g. the Harvard step-test). The heart-rate response to maximal exercise varies with the time of day, though the amplitude is reduced compared to the resting rhythm (Reilly 1990). In many studies of maximal physiological values, it is sometimes uncertain as to whether the ceiling of physiological capability was reached during the exercise test.

The heart-rate responses to submaximal exercise have been used to predict maximal aerobic power (e.g. the Astrand–Ryhming test) and physical working capacity (e.g. the PWC_{150} and PWC_{170} tests). In such tests, heart rates at two or more known submaximal work-rates are either entered into tables to predict oxygen consumption at an estimated maximum heart rate, or used to interpolate a work-rate that elicits a particular heart rate (usually 150–170 beats min^{-1} kcal's min^{-1}). Such tests have been widely adopted for testing large groups of individuals, mainly as part of health education programmes. Although corrections for age and sex have been calculated, these tests still have a large predictive error. Peak-to-trough circadian variations of predicted VO_2 max can be as high as 15% of the 24-hour mean value (Reilly 1990), a finding which is not replicated in studies that have measured VO_2 max directly at different times of the day (see below). A low heart-rate response to exercise produces a high score on these tests. Since the rhythm in heart rate peaks at around 17:00, the acrophase of predicted work capacity may occur 12 hours out of phase with acrophases of body temperature and other performance-related measures (Fig. 4.6). This has led some chronobiologists to the erroneous conclusion that physical performance peaks during the night.

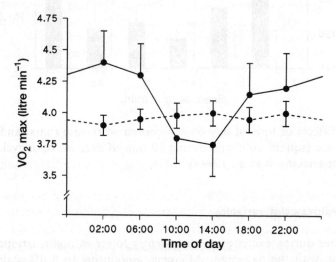

Fig. 4.6 Comparison between circadian variations in predicted (solid line) and directly measured (broken line) $\dot{V}O_2$max (Reilly 1990).

The equation employed in cosinor analysis for determining circadian functions (Chapter 11) can be rearranged to calculate, from known circadian characteristics, the 24-hour mean of a fitness-test score obtained at any time of the solar day:

$$FT_{corr} = \frac{FT_t}{1 + (0.01A \cdot \cos(15t - 15F)} \tag{4.1}$$

where t is the time of day at which the fitness test was measured (decimal clock hours), FT_t is the score for the fitness test at time t, A is the amplitude of the 'standard' rhythm (% of 24-hour mean) and F is the acrophase of the 'standard' rhythm (decimal hours). Circadian data (amplitude, acrophase) from previous studies of the effects of the time of day on fitness tests can be substituted into the above equation to correct the result for time of day. This equation is useful for correcting fitness tests administered to large populations of subjects when it is often not practical to control for the time of day. It is stressed, however, that in order for the above equation to be used, the circadian variation must follow a sinusoidal pattern.

Systolic blood pressure measured before and after set exercise regimens is unaffected by the time of day (Cabri *et al.* 1988). Together with the poor reproducibility associated with sphygmomanometry, the lack of highly controlled pre-exercise conditions may swamp any variations in blood pressure. Despite this, diastolic blood pressure (post-exercise) does vary with time of day; the rhythm reaches an acrophase between 00:00 and 02:00 (Cabri *et al.* 1988). Although the phase of this rhythm is slightly earlier than the normal resting rhythm, it may be that a brief bout of intense effort at night may place unfit individuals with a predisposition towards coronary heart disease at risk of a cardiac event. This 'shock theory' of exercise is supported by the findings of decreased exercise capacity of angina patients in the early morning.

4.4.3 Metabolic parameters

Circadian rhythmicity can be observed in oxygen consumption ($\dot{V}O_2$) at moderate work-rates (150 W) with a peak occurring at about 15:00, but the rhythm can usually be explained fully in terms of circadian variations in bodyweight (Reilly 1990). Significant rhythmicity is evident in $\dot{V}O_2$ responses to a lighter work-rate than 150 W, irrespective of changes in body mass. The time required for $\dot{V}O_2$ to reach steady state (expressed as the value in the fifth minute of exercise) is not usually more than 3 min and does not vary with the time of day. The rhythm in $\dot{V}CO_2$ agrees in phase and amplitude with that of $\dot{V}O_2$. There is therefore, no circadian rhythm in the respiratory exchange ratio (RER) during exercise when dietary intake is highly controlled. Nevertheless, under normal day-to-day living, an athlete's dietary intake is not taken at equally spaced time intervals throughout the solar day. Like everyone else, athletes fast during sleep. Consequently, blood glucose levels tend to be lower in the morning than in the afternoon. Thus, during prolonged exercise in the morning following an overnight fast, RER is lower than in the late afternoon, suggesting that a greater proportion of fatty acids is being used to form ATP (Atkinson *et al.* 1994*b*).

There is a lack of rhythmicity in oxygen consumption during exercise when measured at maximal exercise intensities. In both longitudinal and cross-sectional studies which ensure that the subjects are well motivated to reach exhaustion, it has been found that VO_2 max is a stable function, independent of the time of day of measurement (Reilly 1990). Such a finding is not surprising, since the amplitude of the resting rhythm in $\dot{V}O_2$ if maintained during maximal exercise, would be less than 0.5% $\dot{V}O_2$ max. This small amplitude would be hard to detect given the relative insensitivity of equipment used to measure $\dot{V}O_2$ max.

The rhythm in minute ventilation ($\dot{V}E$) is phased similar to the resting rhythm, but amplified by 20–40% during light or moderate exercise. This rhythm in $\dot{V}E$ is apparent even when expressed as the ventilatory equivalent of oxygen ($\dot{V}E/\dot{V}O_2$) and may explain the reports of mild dyspnoea when exercise is performed in the early morning. Other ventilatory parameters, such as peak expiratory flow and vital capacity of the lungs, are also lowest in the early morning, especially in asthmatics. It is therefore recommended that athletes who suffer from this condition do not exercise before 09:00.

4.5 Physical responses to exercise

The performance components considered in this section are relevant to the safety of exercise. Lack of flexibility or increased stiffness may both play a role in the incidence of sports injuries.

4.5.1 Stature

Human stature is not constant but varies throughout the day. The loss of stature attributed to 'spinal shrinkage' may be important in injury and rehabilitation. Shrinkage refers to the loss of spinal length due to compressive loading; the rest–activity rhythm present in nychthemeral conditions imposes compressive loading on the spine during the day, leading to the extrusion of water through the intervertebral-disc wall and a consequent loss of disc height. This shrinkage is reversed at night during the recumbency of sleeping.

For both male and female subjects, the peak-to-trough variation in stature is 1.1% of the 24-hour mean value. The rhythm is markedly reduced in amplitude in patients with ankylosing spondylitis. A sinusoidal wave provides an unsatisfactory fit to the circadian variation, with the data being better described by a power function (Fig. 4.7). The rhythm is highly exogenous and can be reversed by daytime procedures designed to unload the spine (e.g. the Fowler position in which the subject lies supine with the lower limbs raised about 30 cm above the horizontal). Normally, peak stature occurs after getting out of bed and the minimum is observed just before retiring to bed.

Stature losses in responses to 20 min of weight training are smaller in the evening when body height is in the trough of circadian variation than in the morning (Wilby *et al*. 1987). Greater stiffness of intervertebral discs in the evening may increase the risk of injury, though higher values of back strength in the evening (see above) may compensate for the increase in stiffness. The solution is to ensure that the spine is unloaded by a short period of rest prior to undertaking any strenuous exercise in the evening.

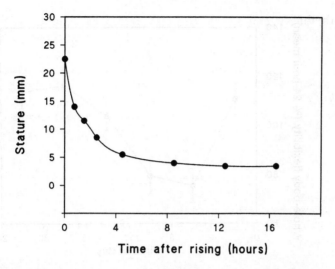

Fig. 4.7 Circadian variation in human stature expressed relative to time after waking. (Reilly 1990). Data are expressed as changes from a reference value on waking.

4.5.2 Flexibility

Joint flexibility (range of movement) shows marked rhythmicity across a wide range of human movements, such as lumbar flexion and extension, glenohumeral lateral rotation and whole-body forward flexion. Amplitudes of these rhythms can be as high as 20% of the 24-hour mean (Fig. 4.8). Values drop to their minimum levels in the morning.

The circadian variation in stiffness (resistance to motion) of the knee joint is similar to that of body temperature, with lowest levels of stiffness being recorded in the early evening (Reilly 1990). However, endogenous mechanisms cannot be fully implicated as the cause of this rhythm because joint stiffness is highly influenced by exogenous factors, such as the amount of prior physical activity.

4.5.3 Other performance-related parameters

The severity of exercise may be gauged by asking the individual to rate it subjectively on a numerical scale. Ratings of perceived exertion (RPE) were found by Faria and Drummond (1982) to be higher during exercise carried out in the early hours of the morning than in the evening. In this study, however, work-rates were set relative to elicited heart rates of 130, 150 and 170 beats min^{-1}. The submaximal heart rate at a set work-rate is lowest at

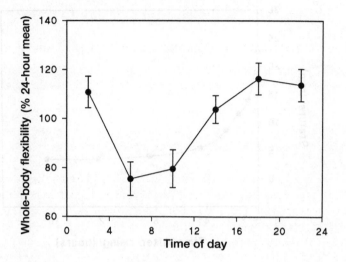

Fig. 4.8 Circadian rhythm in whole-body flexibility measured with a Takei forward flexometer. (Unpublished data obtained from 20 subjects in the laboratory at Liverpool John Moores University.)

night (see above). Thus, the higher subjective ratings reported at this time may have been due to higher exercise intensities and not any circadian variation in RPE. When subjects exercise at levels that are expressed relative to $\dot{V}O_2$ max rather than heart rate, RPE shows a circadian variation but only during high-intensity exercise (Reilly 1990). The RPE scale is based on the response of heart rate to exercise. An increase of 1 in RPE relates to an increment of 10 beats min^{-1} of the heart. Since the circadian variation of heart rate in response to exercise is often less than 10 beats min^{-1}, it is not surprising that fluctuations in RPE are difficult to detect. Heart rate and RPE can also dissociate; low-intensity exercise when performed many times within a solar day may mediate a transient increase in RPE after lunch, without a corresponding increase in submaximal heart rates.

Athletes often experience pain resulting from injuries and discomfort due to extreme competitive exertion. Epicritic pain is localized pain with a relatively high sensitivity. Protopathic pain is diffuse in that it has a relatively low sensitivity. The thresholds for epicritic and protopathic pain both show circadian rhythmicity peaking at 03:00–06:30 and 11:00 respectively (Winget *et al.* 1985). The variation in pain perception appears unrelated to mood states and thus appears to be mediated by endogenous mechanisms. As these circadian rhythms in pain perception are out of phase with rhythms in RPE during exercise, it appears that the mechanisms associated with pain sensation are separate from those concerned with perception of exertion.

4.6 What is the best time of day to train?

Two issues are relevant here which affect the efficacy of a training programme:

1. The time of day at which athletes are prepared voluntarily to work hardest;
2. The time of day which elicits the greatest training responses to standardized exercise regimens.

4.6.1 Habitual circadian variation in the training stimulus

With respect to (1) above, circadian variations in self-selected work-rates have been examined by Atkinson *et al.* (1993*a*) and Coldwells *et al.* (1993). A self-chosen work-rate recorded at the start of 30 minutes of exercise on a cycle ergometer demonstrates rhythmicity with an acrophase at 19:00 and an amplitude of about 7 percent of the 24-hour mean value (Fig. 4.9). The higher work-rates chosen in the evening are not accompanied by any increases in ratings of perceived exertion. This evening preference for higher work-rates may not be apparent when prolonged exercise is performed in hot conditions. Assuming that athletes are exposed to the zeitgebers which are associated with a diurnal existence, it is unlikely that habitual training in the morning over long periods of time (e.g. as carried out by swimmers and gymnasts) would fully reverse the evening superiority of self-selected training stimuli. However, this has not been examined empirically.

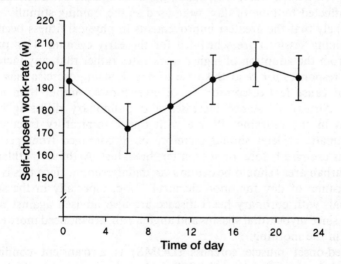

Fig. 4.9 Circadian rhythm in self-selected work-rate. Subjects were asked to pace themselves so that they could sustain the exercise for 30 minutes (Atkinson *et al.* 1993*a*).

4.6.2 Circadian variation in the responses to training

Research on the circadian variation in the efficacy of endurance training programmes is equivocal. In one study, the circadian effects of an aerobic training programme were studied in three groups of men who exercised in either the morning (9:00–9:30), afternoon (15:00–15:30), or evening (20:00–20:30) (Torii *et al.* 1992). Each group cycled for 30 min at 60 percent $\dot{V}O_2$ max (so that the training stimulus was the same, irrespective of time of day) for 4 days per week over a 4-week period. The maximal oxygen uptake ($\dot{V}O_2$ max) was estimated and the adaptive responses of heart rate and blood lactate levels to the training programme were measured. After 4 weeks, the afternoon group showed the greatest increase in estimated $\dot{V}O_2$ max, suggesting that aerobic training is most effective in the afternoon, although $\dot{V}O_2$ and post-training was measured only in the afternoon for the three groups. In addition, other researchers have failed to find any significant differences between the training responses to morning and evening exercise (Hill *et al.* 1989).

Improvements in muscle strength following training sessions scheduled at 21:00 have been reported to be 20% higher than those following training carried out at 09:00 (Gutenbrunner 1993). However, the training stimuli were provided by maximal isometric contractions, which can themselves vary with the time of day. Plasma concentrations of somatotrophin and testosterone were significantly higher following training in the evening compared to the morning (Gutenbrunner 1993); again, maximal muscle contractions, which can be affected by time of day, were used as the training stimuli.

It is likely that the greatest improvements in physical fitness occur when hard training sessions are scheduled for the early evening. This probably results from the adoption of higher work-rates rather than any increases in training responses *per se* at this time of day. Evening exercise may also be safer and cause less discomfort for a given power output than morning exercise. Airway resistance increases and pulmonary diffusing capacity decreases in the morning. People with upper respiratory tract ailments and asthmatic athletes should therefore be discouraged from performing strenuous exercise before, or soon after, breakfast. Asthmatic athletes who train in urban areas should be cautious in midafternoon, since this is usually the peak-time of day for photochemical smog, especially in the summer. Individuals with coronary heart disease are also advised against morning exercise, since myocardial spasms and angina pain are induced more easily by exercise in the morning.

Delayed-onset muscle soreness (DOMS) is a transient condition of musculoskeletal trauma that can follow vigorous exercise, particularly that involving eccentric muscle contractions. Soreness ratings peak 2–3 days after exercise, though any circadian variation within this period has not been researched. The plasma concentration of creatine kinase increases during

DOMS and has been employed as a marker of muscle damage. The lowest ratings of soreness and plasma concentrations of creatine kinase have been found following exercise performed in the evening (Gutenbrunner 1993).

Paradoxically, there is some evidence to suggest that the learning of motor skills is faster when tasks are performed in the early morning, with the greatest improvement occurring in the performance of a pursuit motor task at 09:00 (Gutenbrunner 1993). Further work is still required to replicate this study for skills used specifically in sport and to examine the effect of long-term training in the morning on adaptive responses.

4.7 Individual differences in performance rhythms

Individual differences in preferred sleep-times were recognized in the nineteenth century. In the following sections, interindividual differences in circadian performance characteristics are discussed.

4.7.1 Chronotype

The classification of morning-types ('larks'), evening-types ('owls') and intermediate-types (neither larks nor owls) is based on the responses to questions regarding sleep and waking times and the phasing of work and habitual activity (Chapter 1). The acrophase of the rhythm in oral temperature occurs slightly earlier in larks compared to owls. Scores on the 'morningness' questionnaire are a better predictor of body-temperature phase than sleep and waking times *per se*, suggesting that chronotype is not just dependent on the phase of the sleep–wake cycle. Phase advances in 'larks' have also been reported for rhythms in subjective alertness and adrenaline secretion.

With respect to human performance in industrial contexts, performance (measured as the correct rejection of faulty items on a production line) is significantly better in the morning for 'larks' compared to 'owls', and *vice versa* during evening work. Post-lunch dips in performance seem to be more pronounced in morning-types. The results of studies that have examined chronotype differences in exercise performance are not so conclusive. The responses to exercise (100 W and a work-rate corresponding to maximal oxygen consumption) on a cycle ergometer were compared between morning-type and evening-types by Hill *et al.* (1988). The results of this study showed that diurnal variations in submaximal heart rate, perceived exertion, and oxygen consumption were not affected by subject chronotype. This research group reported that the highest possible oxygen consumption in evening-types occurred in the evening, whereas the highest oxygen consumption achieved by morning-types was not related to the time of day. Motivational factors may have played a role in this latter observation, since it is unusual to find an effect of time of day on directly measured maximal oxygen consumption with well-motivated subjects.

Examinations of chronotypes among athletic populations are rare and the results are difficult to interpret. It is unclear whether athletes with certain chronotypes gravitate towards certain sports that are scheduled at their most preferable time, or that athletes become accustomed to the time of day at which certain events are held. 'Morningness – eveningness questionnaires have been given to golfers, whose competing time varied with the time of day, and water-polo players, who performed mostly in the evening (Rossi *et al.* 1983). The elite golfers in the experimental sample showed higher scores for 'morningness' than the water-polo players. 'Morningness' is higher than usual in cycling time-triallists, especially veteran competitors aged over 40 years (Atkinson *et al.* 1994*a*). These athletes often compete very early in the morning.

4.7.2 Personality

Although personality seems to have an effect on sleep-times (introverts get up earlier in the day), there is no convincing evidence of a relationship between introversion or extroversion and either chronotype or circadian rhythms in body temperature and performance (Kerkof 1985). Chronotype may be more influenced by traits of personality other than extroversion or introversion. For example, psychologically stable introverts possess high heart rates in the early part of the day, while neurotic introverts show high heart rates in the evening.

4.7.3 Sex

Females have been found to have higher mean body temperatures than males over a 24-hour period than males (Winget *et al.* 1985), and smaller rhythm amplitudes in body temperature. Peak temperature also occurs later in the solar day in females, while the minimum occurs earlier. There appears to be no research work on gender differences in circadian performance rhythms. Such work should control for the phase of the menstrual cycle, a factor which has been overlooked in previous studies involving females subjects. Body temperature is increased during the luteal phase of the menstrual cycle.

4.7.4 Physical fitness or activity level

The rhythm amplitudes in body temperature, arousal, and performance variables of physically fit subjects are around 1.5 times higher than in unfit individuals, when studied under standardized laboratory conditions (Harma *et al.* 1982; Atkinson *et al.* 1993*b*). The greater rhythm amplitude in body temperature for physically fit subjects is accounted for by a minimum that is 0.4 °C lower than in the unfit subjects (Fig. 4.10). Although exercise during the day increases body temperature, there is a proportional drop in body temperature after exercise below the temperature observed during 'normal' sleep (sleep following no activity during the day). This 'post-exercise thermoregulatory overcompensation' (Mermin and Czeisler 1987) cannot explain the rhythm differences between fit and unfit subjects since, in the above studies, rhythms were compared under controlled conditions with a random order of testing. This implies that the lower nocturnal body temperatures of physically fit subjects may be mediated via endogenous mechanisms (a training effect of habitual physical activity or rhythm characteristics peculiar to athletes). It is plausible that there is an influence of the documented sleep characteristics of athletes. There is generally an increase in 'slow-wave sleep' and sleep length in athletes which are, in turn, associated with lower body temperature during sleep.

4.7.5 Age

Circadian timing is altered in elderly individuals. This applies to circadian rhythms in body temperature, hormonal secretions, haematological parameters, and the urinary excretion of metabolites. Rhythms with a large exogenous component, such as heart rate and blood pressure, are also different in elderly individuals, although probably as a consequence of changes in the sleep–wake cycle and the cardiovascular responses to meals (Atkinson *et al.* 1994*c*). The most consistent age-related circadian differences are a reduction in the amplitudes or a 'flattening' of the rhythms, as well as a rise in the variability of rhythm acrophases. Rhythm acrophases of elderly subjects often occur earlier than normal in the solar day, in agreement with other observations of earlier wake–times and increased 'morningness' in old age (Fig. 4.11). Veteran cyclists seem more likely to be morning-type individuals, scheduling greater amounts of training before 14:00 than young adults. This is evident before the older cyclists have retired from work (Atkinson *et al.* 1994*a*). The performance of veteran cyclists in time-trials is also less affected by early morning starts. Laboratory studies have confirmed that, although subjects aged 50–60 years still perform best in the early evening, they also perform relatively well in the morning, with age-differences in performance being least at this time (Atkinson *et al.* 1992; Atkinson *et al.* 1994*b*). It is still unclear whether such findings reflect age-related changes in the endogenous clock or exogenous influences such as sleep.

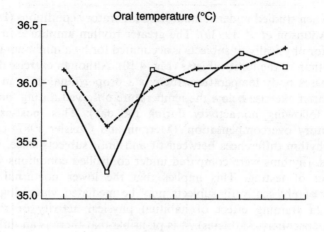

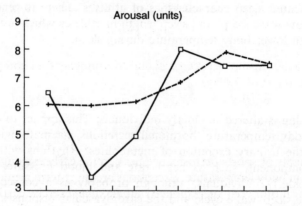

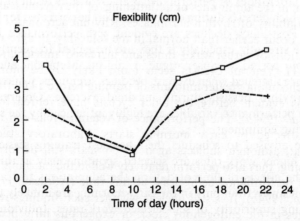

Fig. 4.10 Comparison of circadian rhythms between physically fit (solid line) and unfit (broken line) subjects (Atkinson *et al.*, 1993*b*).

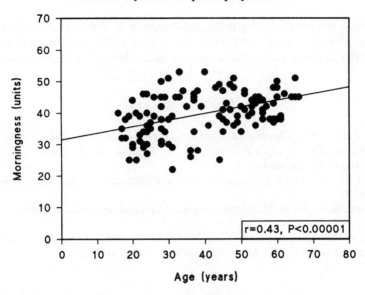

Fig. 4.11 The relationship between age and 'morningness' in competitive cyclists (Atkinson *et al.* 1994a).

4.8 Overview

Most components of sports performance peak in the early evening, close to the maximum in body temperature. Exceptions are short-term memory, tasks demanding fine motor control, prolonged submaximal exercise carried out in hot conditions, and predictive tests of physical fitness, which all peak in the morning. The latter index of performance is an erroneous result of the heart-rate rhythm, which persists during exercise and can be corrected for by means of equations. Post-lunch declines are evident with performance variables, such as muscle strength, especially if they are measured frequently enough within a 24-hour period to cause fatigue in subjects. Metabolic and respiratory rhythms are flattened when exercise becomes strenuous, while the body-temperature rhythm persists during maximal exercise. Observations of rhythmicity in performance variables are highly influenced by the sensitivity of the measuring equipment.

Athletes are advised to schedule their heaviest training session in the evening since higher work-rates are selected spontaneously at this time of day, though the effects of time of day on the adaptations to training are unclear. Athletes who train only in the early morning are unlikely to reverse fully the evening superiority of self-selected work-rates. Individual differences in performance rhythms are small, but significant. Although most athletes perform best in a 'window' or about 3–4 hours on either side of their peakbody temperature, the minute differences in ability that exist between the winners and runners-up mean that subtle differences in rhythm characteristics between competitors may considerably affect athletic success.

Further reading

Monk T. H. (1992). Chronobiology of mental performance. In *Biological rhythms in clinical and laboratory medicine* (ed. Y. Touitou and E. Haus), pp. 208–13. Springer-Verlag, Berlin.
Reilly T. (1990). Human circadian rhythms and exercise. *Crit. Rev. Biomed. Eng.*, **18**, 165–80.
Shephard, R. J. (1984). Sleep, biorhythms and human performance. *Sports Med.*, **1**, 11–37.
Winget C. M., Deroshia C. W., and Holley D. C. (1985). Circadian rhythms and athletic performance. *Med. Sci. Sports Exerc.* **17**, 498–516.

References

Atkinson, G., Coldwells, A., Reilly, T., and Waterhouse, J. (1992). An age-comparison of circadian rhythms in physical performance and mood states. *J. Interdisciplin. Cycle Res.* **23**, 186–8.
Atkinson, G., Coldwells, A., Reilly, T., and Waterhouse, J. (1993*a*) Circadian rhythmicity in self-chosen work-rate. In *Chronobiology and chronomedicine. Basic research and applications* (ed. C. Gutenbrunner, G. Hildebrandt, and R. Moog), pp. 478–84. Lang-Verlag, Frankfurt.
Atkinson, G., Coldwells, A., Reilly, T., and Waterhouse, J. (1993*b*). A comparison of circadian rhythms in work performance between physically active and inactive subjects. *Ergonomics*, **36**, 273–81.
Atkinson, G., Coldwells A., Reilly T., and Waterhouse J. (1994*a*). The influence of age on diurnal variations in competitive cycling performances (abstr.). *J. Sports Sci.*, **12**, 127.
Atkinson, G., Coldwells A., Reilly T., and Waterhouse J. (1994*b*). Effects of age on diurnal variations in prolonged physical performance and the physiological responses to exercise (abstr.). *J. Sports Sci.*, **12**, 127.
Atkinson G., Witte K., Nold G., Sasse U., and Lemmer B. (1994c). Effects of age on circadian blood pressure and heart rate rhythms in patients with primary hypertension. *Chronobiol. Int.*, **11**, 35–44.
Baxter, C. and Reilly, T. (1983). Influence of time of day on all-out swimniing, *Brit. J. Sports Med.*, **17**, 122–7.
Cabri, J., Clarys, J. P., De Witte, B., Reilly, T., and Strass, D. (1988). Circadian variation in blood pressure responses to muscular exercise. *Ergonomics*, **31**, 1559–66.
Coldwells, A., Atkinson, G., Reilly, T., and Waterhouse, J. (1993). Self-chosen work-rate determines day–night differences in work capacity (abstr.). *Ergonomics*, **36**, 313.

Faria, I. E. and Drummond, B. J. (1982). Circadian changes in resting heart rate and body temperature, maximal oxygen consumption and perceived exertion. *Ergonomics*, **25**, 381–6.

Gutenbrunner, C. H. R. (1993). Circadian variations of physical training. In *Chronobiology and chronomedicine: basic research and applications* (ed. C. Gutenbrunner, G. Hildebrandt, and R. Moog), pp. 665–80. Lang–Verlag. Frankfurt.

Harkness, J. A., Richter, M. B., Panagi, G. S., Van de Pete, K., Linger, A., Pownall, R., and Geddawi, M. (1982). Circadian variation in disease activity in rheumatoid arthritis, *Brit. Med. J.*, **284**, 551–5.

Harma, M. I., Ilmarinen, J. and Yletyiner, I. (1982). Circadian variation of physiological functions in physically average and very fit dayworkers. *J. Hum. Ergol.*, **11**, Suppl. 1, 33–46.

Hessemer, V., Langusch, D., Bruck, K., Bodeker, R. K., and Breidenbach, T. (1984). Effects of slightly lowered body temperature on endurance performance in humans. *J. Appl. Physiol. Resp. Environ. Exer. Physiol.*, **57**, 1731–7.

Hill, D. W., Cureton, K. J., Collins, M. A., and Gresham, S. C. (1988). Diurnal variations in responses to exercise of 'morning types' and 'evening types'. *J. Sports Med. Phys. Fit.*, **28**, 213–19.

Hill, D. W., Cureton, K. J., and Collins, M. A. (1989). Circadian specificity in exercise training. *Ergonomics*, **32**, 79–92.

Kerkof, G. (1985). Individual differences in circadian rhythms. In *Hours of work: temporal factors in work scheduling* (ed. S. Folkard and T. Monk), pp. 29–35. Wiley, Chichester.

Mermin, J. and Czeisler, C. (1987). Comparison of ambulatory temperature recordings at varying levels of physical exertion: average amplitude is unchanged by strenuous exercise. *Sleep Res.*, **16**, 253 (Abstract).

Reilly, T. (1990). Human circadian rhythms and exercise. *Crit. Rev. Biomed. Eng.*, **18**, 165–80.

Reilly, T. and Brooks, G. A. (1986). Exercise and the circadian variation in body temperature measures. *Int. J. Sports Med.*, **7**, 358–62.

Reilly, T. and Down, A. (1986). Circadian variation in the standing broad jump. *Percept. Motor Skills*, **62**, 830.

Reilly, T. and Marshall S. (1991). Circadian rhythms in power output on a swim bench. *J. Swim. Res.* **7**, 11–13.

Rossi, B., Zani A., and Mecacci L. (1983). Diurnal individual differences and performance levels in some sports activities. *Percept. Motor Skills*, **57**, 27–30.

Torii, J., Shinkai, S., Hino, S., Kurokawa, Y., Tomita, M., Watanabe, S., and Watanabe, T. (1992). Effect of time of day on adaptive response to a 4-week aerobic exercise program. *J. Sports Med. Phys. Fit.*, **32**, 348–52.

Wilby, J., Linge, K., Reilly, T., and Troup, J. D. G. (1987). Spinal shrinkage in females: circadian variation and the effects of circuit weight-training. *Ergonomics*, **30**, 47–54.

Winget, C. M., Deroshia, C. W., and Holley, D. C. (1985). Circadian rhythms and athletic performance. *Med. Sci. Sports Exerc.* **17**, 498–516.

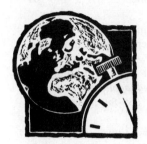

5
Sleep and exercise

5.1 Introduction

One of the more fundamental human circadian rhythms is the sleep–wakefulness cycle. While asleep, the organism is virtually unresponsive to external stimuli; this is in sharp contrast with a state of extreme alertness. In this sense, the states associated with the sleep–wakefulness cycle constitute a continuum from deep sleep to high excitement. The biphasic rhythm in human lives is in most cases matched to the light and dark cycles in the environment caused by the rotation of the earth around its long axis.

The activities of animals and birds are organized on either a diurnal or nocturnal basis. These patterns are teleological and determine the feeding, foraging, and resting routines that ensure the survival of the species. Humans are geared for a diurnal cycle, and on average one-third of human life is spent asleep. The implications of the sleep–wakefulness cycle for mental performance have been covered in Chapter 3 and the consequences of shifting to a nocturnal pattern of work are described in Chapter 8.

The duration is not the only characteristic of a good night's sleep. Other important aspects are restfulness, as indicated by relative movements, and latency, which is indicated according to some researchers by the time between lights-out and the onset of Stage 2 sleep. The average length of sleep is about 8 hours, but there is a large variation between individuals both in the amount taken (the coefficient of variation is approximately 30%) and in that needed for effective well-being.

To some extent sleep is an enigma, and a complete understanding of sleep is still beyond the scope of current clinical means of assessing it. We take sleep for granted and, apart from exceptional cases of chronic insomnia, it is assumed to be essential for normal restorative biological processes. The capacity of sleep to restore well-being is acknowledged in Shakespeare's *Macbeth*:

> 'Sleep that knits up the ravell'd sleave of care,
> The death of each day's life, sore labour's bath,
> Balm of hurt minds, great nature's second course,
> Chief nourisher in life's feast.'

5.2 Sleep stages

5.2.1 REM and nonREM sleep

Sleep is not a single lengthy slump in 'slumberland' but is comprised of a series of sleep stages (Fig. 5.1). Each stage exhibits characteristic waveforms on the electroencephalograph (EEG), computer-aided analysis of which has helped enormously in understanding the underlying events. The two major types of sleep are:

1. Rapid eye movement (REM) sleep, which comprises about 20% of total sleep. It is discernible by electro-oculography (EOG), as the eyes flick from side to side beneath closed eyelids for periods of several minutes at a time.
2. The remaining nonREM sleep, which is subdivided into Stages 1 to 4.

In nonREM sleep, stages 3 and 4 together are referred to as slow-wave sleep because of the high-amplitude, low-frequency EEG waves associated with them. Stage 2 occupies a greater duration than any of the other stages and usually precedes or follows REM sleep, the phase in which dreaming takes place. The REM pattern appears predominantly in the latter part of the entire sleep period, while Stage 4 occurs mainly in the early part. REM occurs regularly about five or six times during each sleep period. The periodicity of about 90 min has given rise to the supposition that an internal ultradian oscillator is involved in the generation of REM sleep.

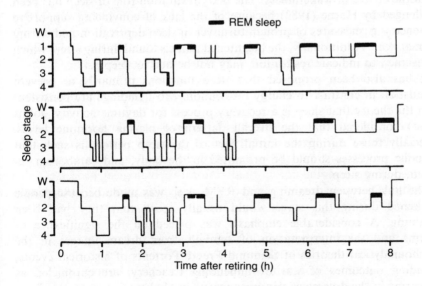

Fig. 5.1 Characteristic stages of a normal night's sleep on three consecutive nights.

Significant 90–100 min oscillations are linked with ultradian rhythms in cognitive style in the daytime; this supports the hypothesis that the basic rest–activity cycle in humans involves alternating the activation of different processing systems residing in the two cerebral hemispheres. The EEG waveform of REM sleep closely resembles that of daytime drowsiness. It is possible that the periodicity may continue throughout the nychthemeron (or everyday conditions) since it seems to be an integral aspect of neuronal organization. As this rhythm would affect daytime levels of arousal, it has speculatively been linked with the paradoxical drop in mental and physical performance often reported for midafternoon when body temperature is still rising and approaching its highest point. This has been referred to elsewhere as the 'post-lunch dip'.

5.2.2 Role of sleep stages

NonREM sleep is thought to be directed towards body restitution, while REM sleep associated with increases in cerebral synthetic processes, including a high rate of brain-protein synthesis and the consolidation of memory traces. The body-restitution theory is based on the observation of elevated levels of growth hormone in plasma during slow-wave sleep (Adam and Oswald 1977); protein synthesis for tissue restoration is thought to accelerate while the powerhouses of the cell, the mitochondria, recover at nighttime from the effects of wakefulness. The body-restitution role of sleep has been challenged by Horne (1983) because of the lack of convincing supportive evidence, e.g. measures of protein turnover in sleep deprivation and during normal sleep. Additionally, the heightened mitosis found during sleep, which is assumed to indicate restitution, may not be due to sleep *per se*.

It has also been proposed that sleep functions primarily to prevent exhaustion in contrast to energy restoration. Most findings are consistent with the theory that sleep is a recovery process for daytime activity. Johns (1981) considered that the overall pattern of plasma hormone levels, especially those during the initial part of the sleep period, is such that anabolic processes should be promoted in the body, and catabolism reduced, during sleep.

The link between dreaming and REM sleep was made because people awakened during this stage would usually recall that they had been dreaming. A considerable emphasis was placed on the significance of dreams and the interpretation of symbols from dream images in the psychoanalytical theories of Sigmund Freud. Portents of historical events, including outcomes of war or impending treachery, are chronicled as appearing in the dreams of the protagonists in Shakespearean drama. Such links between dreams and reality are not substantiated by the work of contemporary sleep researchers.

5.3 Sleep and circadian rhythms

Sleep is affected by the circadian oscillator. In free-running experiments, the time of sleep onset occurs most frequently near the time of the body-temperature trough. The duration of sleep depends on when in the circadian cycle sleep is initiated; the later the individual goes to bed, the shorter the duration of sleep is likely to be.

Sleep is intimately related to the circadian rhythm in arousal; together, the two rhythms constitute the sleep–wakefulness cycle. Since melatonin production by the pineal gland is entrained and suppressed by light, it is thought that this hormone and its precursors have important roles in the regulation of sleep. Melatonin levels are typically 10 times higher in plasma samples taken during the night compared to daytime values. The rhythm is highly reproducible for any individual but is disturbed in patients with sleep disorders. There are as yet no wholly satisfactory mechanistic explanations of how sleep is regulated.

There is a rich history of research into sleep substances and how their active ingredients might modulate sleep behaviour. This is likely to depend on the specific sleep-enhancing action of each substance, the time of day, the irregularity of many sleep factors, and the feedback regulation of sleep-waking states (Inoue 1989). In addition, some of these many substances have shown interactions between slow-wave sleep and the immune system (Fig. 5.2). The hypothalamus and raphe system are linked not only with sleep regulation, but also with immune function and temperature regulation. Clearly, the control system governing sleep requires a highly complex integration of neuronal, physiological and cellular mechanisms, including how they operate in the human brain.

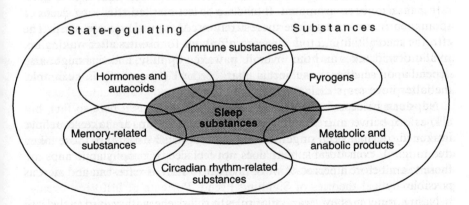

Fig. 5.2 A schematic representation of the involvement of multiple humoral factors in the regulation of sleep (Inoue 1989).

5.4 The role of naps

It is not unusual for adults, particularly elderly ones, to nap during the daytime, but it seems that all subjects benefit from naps during prolonged work-hours and as a means of catching up on lost sleep. Thus, a 2-hour nap after a vigil of 45 hours or 53 hours results in a considerable degree of recuperation and a 4-hour nap substantially reverses the decrement during the daytime that would normally follow a night without sleep. A 1-hour nap taken at 02:00 during a night without sleep was reported to reduce the overnight decrement in auditory vigilance, but not in more complex visual vigilance and logical-thought tests (Naitoh 1981).

Since there are many types of mental performance, and their rates of decrement vary with increasing duration of performance, it is not surprising that not all decrements appear to be reversed, or reduced, equally easily. Even so, there have been attempts to see if more frequent, shorter naps are as effective as less frequent, longer ones. Put differently, is our 8-hour/16-hour sleep/active day the ideal, or would two equal 12-hour 'days' (4 hours/8 hours, sleep/active), or even shorter days (involving multiple sleeps each of 2 hours, 1 hour, or even 20 minutes) be equally effective? In one sense, the shorter the day, the less decrement there is in mental performance. This result presumably reflects the fact that performance – particularly in very repetitive or complex tasks or in those requiring vigilance – falls off with time spent on a particular task.

There is, however, another effect of naps that tends to offset the advantage of many short sleeps; this is 'sleep inertia'. It is the phenomenon whereby, immediately after waking from a nap, particularly one during the night, performance *falls* for some minutes after being woken. The effect seems to be more marked if the subject wakes from slow-wave sleep and/or in a quiet rather than noisy environment. It tends to be less marked after long sleeps or spontaneous awakening since these rarely occur from slow-wave sleep. The effect is generally found to have worn off about 10 minutes after waking up. In addition, it takes an hour or more to waken up fully; and this might also depend upon whether the subject is a 'lark' or 'owl' (Chapter 1). For example, the latter have more difficulty in the morning.

Naps can be described as 'recuperative' (the sense used here so far), but also as 'appetitive' and 'prophylactic'. Recuperative naps are taken to relieve fatigue due to lost sleep or activity, or both; appetitive naps are those taken due to habit, even if the subject does not feel sleepy; prophylactic naps are those taken before a period of work in order to start as refreshed and alert as possible.

Naps appear to obey very similar rules to full sleeps, with regard to the ease of initiating sleep and its composition. However, brief naps will be too short to allow slow-wave sleep to be reached, and so contain mainly Stage 2 sleep. It can be seen that taking naps, while a very effective way of reducing performance decrement, might be an *inefficient* way of doing so if they are too brief. Accepting that sleep loss might occur, it is also appropriate to note that a marked deterioration in performance of a vigilance test did not occur in a group of subjects until their regular sleep duration at night had been reduced from 8 hours to 5.5 hours (Stampi *et al.* 1990). This can be interpreted to indicate that we normally sleep longer than necessary and this would fit in with the concept of dividing sleep into obligatory and facultative portions, the optional (facultative) part coming second in a normal night.

5.5 Complete sleep loss

Many individuals who have suffered a complete loss of sleep for two consecutive nights experience temporary visual hallucinations. Most people have such an experience by the third night without sleep. At this time, behaviour becomes bizarre, and psychotic-like symptoms are often displayed. In such circumstances, it is very difficult to sustain meaningful physical exercise without risk of error. Changes in mental states reflect alterations in biochemical and neurotransmitter activities within the brain. For example, it is likely that phenylethylamine, a naturally occurring amine in the brain, may play a role in these cycles of behaviours and mood. By the third night of complete sleep deprivation, urinary levels of this substance approach the values normally observed in psychiatric patients (Reilly 1990). Individuals experiencing such trances may be abruptly snapped out of them if their companions provide strong verbal encouragement to keep awake.

Sleep loss interacts with circadian rhythms, in that the adverse effects of sleep deprivation are most keenly noted at nighttime. In self-paced work sustained for 3–4 days, the activity level peaks at about 18:00, coinciding with the peak of body temperature. This peak persists for as many days as the individual can be kept awake (Fig. 5.3). The effects of 3–4 days of complete sleep loss can be seen as a trend to deteriorating performance on which a circadian rhythm is superimposed. The trend is not evident in all functions; gross motor functions, such as muscle strength, are highly resistant to the effects of sleep loss, while cognitive functions are easily affected.

Complex and challenging mental tasks are less affected than monotonous or boring ones. Strong motivation can often override the effects of sleep loss. If the task is prolonged, it will become progressively more difficult to maintain the required level.

Sleep loss and environmental factors interact, but not in a predictable or additive manner: for example, heat, compounds the effects of loss of sleep, while noise tends partly to offset them. Individual expectations and previous experience of sleep deprivation may also be relevant. Clearly, it is not easy to ascertain the interplay of the various factors affecting performance after sleep loss.

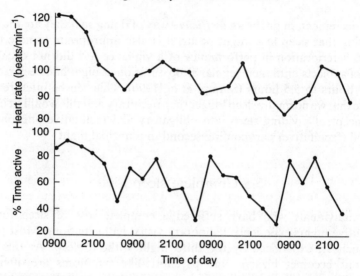

Fig. 5.3 The mean heart rate and the percentage of time active, as measured every 4 hours in four outfield "indoor soccer" players. The recordings for heart rate lagged behind those for activity by 1 hour. The horizontal axis indicates successive days of play (Reilly 1994, p. 240).

Such extreme losses of sleep are rarely met in normal clinical practice, but they may be experienced by sports medical personnel on hospital duty. They may also be encountered for a single night by those participating in 24-hour sports events. Military recruits may be exposed to more than one night in succession without sleep as part of their training. Even longer periods must be faced during charity sports activities that attempt to set unofficial endurance records. The activity levels of footballers playing without sleep or rest for four complete days shows a circadian rhythm (Fig. 5.3). A drop in performance is much more evident in reaction time, due to its neural component (Fig. 5.4). Exercise itself has a powerful arousing effect, and is a good antidote to sleepiness.

The ebb and flow of arousal levels that is characteristic of circadian rhythmicity is evident under sleep-loss conditions. Fatigue and the loss of vigour increase progressively each night and more effort is needed each day to maintain performance in standard laboratory tests. Each successive day of sleep loss is characterized by elevations in the daytime peaks of adrenaline and noradrenaline. These peaks coincide with the high-point of rifle-shooting performance (Froberg *et al.* 1972) as illustrated in Fig. 5.5.

5.6 Partial sleep loss

Most sports coaches consider a good night's sleep is of paramount impor-tance for the athlete, especially during the night before competition. This belief extends to sports spectators, as shown by supporters of the Brazilian soccer team, who created a disturbance outside the residence of the English team on the night before the two countries met in the 1970 World Cup in Mexico. The England Rugby Union team had a similar experience prior to one of its games in the 1995 World Cup in South Africa. There have been many other examples, particularly at the 'athlete's villages' of major tournaments. The tenet is difficult to test since athletes are understandably reluctant to forego or disrupt sleep for experimental reasons, though sedentary subjects have volunteered in abundance for sleep-deprivation studies of less arduous performances.

For the travelling sports-competitor, partial sleep loss is a more common problem than total sleep deprivation. Although there is a large variability in the amount of sleep normally taken by adults, most athletes are convinced that they need a good night's sleep if they are to perform well. This is commonly understood to mean 8 hours of uninterrupted sleep. Sports competitors accept uncritically the need for good sleeping habits, despite many examples of colleagues who cope well with athletic engagements after a poor night's sleep.

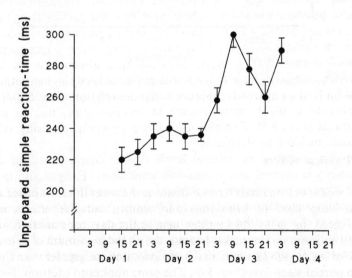

Fig. 5.4 It Unprepared simple reaction-time measured every 4 hours while subjects were playing soccer indoors for 4 days. Mean values ($\pm$SD) are shown (Reilly 1994, p. 250).

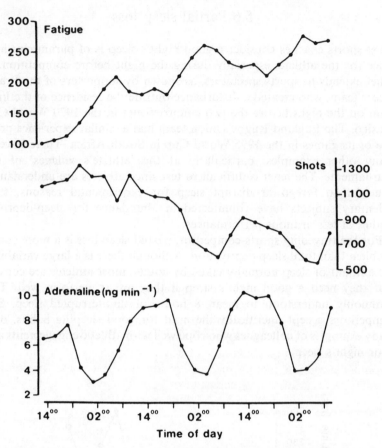

Fig. 5.5 Circadian rhythm in catecholamines, arousal, and shooting performance over successive days of sleep deprivation (Froberg *et al.* 1972).

5.6.1 Physical effects

There appears to be no difference between the sexes in terms of responses to partial sleep loss. In both men and women, adverse effects are most pronounced in tasks demanding neuromuscular coordination, and less marked in gross motor tasks. Indeed, the circadian variation in the performance of tasks such as a maximal hand grip, is much greater than the change due to partial sleep loss (Fig. 5.6). The same applies to exertion, such as all-out swims over 100 m or 400 m (Sinnerton and Reilly 1992).

5.6.2 Mental effects

Disrupted sleep can promote anxiety in those who believe that good-quality sleep is essential. Coordination tasks seem to be more easily affected than gross motor task, such as running, cycling, or exerting maximal muscle tension. This assumes that the individuals concerned are strongly motivated to perform at their maximum. Weight-training exercises may be unaffected by partial sleep loss early on in a training session, but the performance suffers due to lack of drive and concentration as the session continues. The drop in quality of training has been linked with deteriorations in mood with successive nights of sleep disruption (Reilly and Piercy 1994).

5.6.3 Dealing with sleep loss

Individuals forced to reduce their normal sleep ration may adapt to their new regimen without any obvious consequences for performance, provided the reduction does not exceed 2 h. Otherwise, they may need to reorganize their daily routine to accommodate an afternoon nap. There has been no substantive research on the refreshing effects of napping on subsequent exercise performance. Advocacy of a nap for athletes prior to competition would depend on factor, such as timing of the contest, precompetition feeding, and individual preferences.

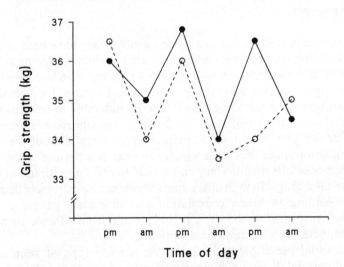

Fig. 5.6 Grip strength measured in the morning and evening in subjects with restricted sleep and after normal sleep (Reilly and Hales 1988).

5.7 Sleeplessness

5.7.1 Insomnia

True insomnia (i.e. complete sleeplessness) is rare, but there are many people, perhaps 10–15 per cent of the population, who have difficulty sleeping. Causes include anxiety, depression, bereavement, stress, overwork, and environmental noise, such as that from motor vehicles or loud music. Some of these problems are transient and selflimiting; others may persist and become chronic.

It is generally thought that exercise promotes sleep, and so regular bouts of physical activity are recommended as therapy for individuals who are having difficulty in sleeping. The effect of exercise is likely to be indirect, with sleep being promoted because exercise has helped to alleviate the anxieties that prevented it. Athletes exhibit different sleep patterns from those of their sedentary peers according to electroencephalographic (EEG) observations. However, EEG characteristics are only marginally altered by a regimen of physical training (Reilly 1986). Strenuous exercise shortly before retiring to sleep is likely to raise the level of arousal rather than induce drowsiness, due to an increase in circulating catecholamine and metabolite levels. Thus, if exercise therapy is prescribed for sleeping problems, it should not be strenuous, and it should be performed early, rather than late, in the evening.

5.7.2 Sleeping pills

People often claim that they need a 'sleeping pill' if they have been unable to sleep at all during the previous night. Such accounts may be untrue and need independent corroboration. Short periods of sleep, snatched unwittingly during the night, provide a significant restorative function. Individuals who manage without sleep for some time derive considerable benefit from such naps, and those deprived of sleep for 2–4 days usually recover from their ordeal after one complete night of uninterrupted sleep. One of the benozdiazepines, temazapam, has been widely misused as a 'leisure' drug. It has been used in cocktails with Ecstacy and 'crack' to offset the stimulant effects of these 'leisure' drugs. In high doses, temazapam can be extremely damaging to health, leading to blood coagulation and ultimately gangrene. Legal crackdown on misuse of the drug in 1995 made it an offence to possess temazapam without a doctor's prescription.

A more usual prescription for insomnia is some type of sleeping pill. People taking sedatives or hypnotics for a prolonged period become dependent upon them, and the drugs progressively lose their effectiveness. The minor tranquillizers, the benzodiazepines, are probably now being overprescribed as treatment for anxiety, both in Europe and in North America. Habitual users of benzodiazepines also become dependent and suffer severe withdrawal symptoms when the drug is no longer prescribed. The dosage levels normally prescribed impair reaction-time and reduce mental concentration the morning after the medication is taken. The same applies to all-out muscular efforts which may be impaired by a hangover effect of the slow-acting drugs of this type (Reilly 1996). Consequently, short-acting hypnotics may be preferred as a method of inducing sleep.

5.7.3 Other means

Hypnotherapy is one nonpharmacological method of treating sleeplessness quite effectively. Biofeedback of skin resistance and EEG signals may also be employed to induce relaxation, thus training individuals to overcome the emotional tension that keeps them awake. Psychological techniques, such as visualization of tranquil scenes, concentration on relaxing muscle activity, and deep breathing, provide alternative methods of treatment. Stimulus-control therapy refers to a mental strategy whereby bed and sleeplessness are dissociated; the individual goes to bed only when sleepy, avoids eating, reading, or watching television in the bedroom, and does not 'sleep in' during the morning. Sensible eating and drinking habits (e.g. avoiding large meals, heavy alcoholic beverages, or caffeine late at night) also promote sleep, and so help rid the patient of problems with sleeplessness.

5.8 Overview

Phenomena associated with sleep will continue to intrigue researchers. These include the interpretation of dreams, sleep walking, and talking during sleep. There is currently an intensive body of research projects concerned with clinical conditions, such as sleep apnoea, and neuronal mechanisms related to sleep-dependent changes in autonomic function. Although some progress has been made in understanding the relationship between exercise and sleep, there are many questions still to be answered. So far, research has not led to a consensus of opinion about the essential role of sleep nor the degree to which its loss impinges on exercise capacity. There are many methodological and ethical issues in the design of research studies on sleep and exercise. The difficulties and constraints should serve as a challenge rather than a deterrent to researchers eager to augment the established facts about the intricate web of relationships between exercise and sleep.

Further reading

Colquhoun, W. P. (ed.). (1971). *Biological rhythms and human performance*. Cambridge University Press, Cambridge.

Horne, J. A. (1988). *Why we sleep: the function of sleep in humans and other mammals*. Oxford University Press.

Reilly, T. (1990). Time zone shifts and sleep deprivation problems. In *Current therapy in sports medicine*, No. 2, (ed. J. S. Torg, R. I. Welsh, and R. J. Shephard), pp. 135–8. Decker, Toronto.

References

Adam, K. and Oswald, I. (1977). Sleep is for tissue restitution. *J. Roy. Coll. Physicians*, 376–88.

Froberg, J. *et al.* (1972). Circadian variations in performance, psychological ratings, catecholamine excreation and diuresis during prolonged sleep deprivation. *Intnal J. Psychol.*, **2**, 23–36.

Horne, J. A. (1983). Human sleep and tissue restitution: some qualifications and doubts. *Clin. Sci.*, **65**, 569–78.

Inoue, S. (1989). *Biology of sleep substances*. In: CRC Press, Boca Reton, Florida.

Johns, M. W. (1981). Sleep. In *The principles and practice of human physiology* (ed. O. G. Edholm and J. S. Weiner). Academic Press, London.

Naitoh, P. (1981). Circadian cycles and the restorative power of naps. *In Biological rhythms, sleep and shift work* (ed. L. Johnson, D. Tepas, W. Colquhoun, and M. Colligan), pp.553–80. Spectrum, New York.

Reilly, T. (1986). Sleep and exercise: an overview. In *Sports science* (ed. J. Watkins, T. Reilly and L. Burwitz), pp. 414–15. Spon, London.

Reilly, T. (1994). Circadian rhythms. In *Oxford textbook of sports medicine* (ed. M. Harries, C. Williams, W. D. Stanish, and L. J. Micheli), pp. 238–54. Oxford University Press, New York.

Reilly, T. (1996). Alcohol, anti-anxiety drugs and sport. In *Drugs in sport*, (2nd edn) (ed. D. R. Mottram), pp. 144–72. Spon, London.

Reilly, T. and Hales, A. J. (1988). Effects of partial sleep deprivation on performance measures in females. In *Contemporary ergonomics 1988* (ed. E. D. Megaw), pp.509–14. Taylor and Francis, London.

Reilly, T. and Piercy, M. (1994). The effect of partial sleep deprivation in weight-lifting performance. *Ergonomics*, **37**, 106–15.

Sinnerton, S. and Reilly, T. (1992). Effects of sleep loss and time of day in swimmers. In Biomechanics and medicine in swimming: swimming science VI (ed. D. MacLaren, T. Reilly, and A. Lees), pp.399–404 Spon, London.

Stampi, C., Broughton R., Mullington, J., Rivers, M, and Campos, J. (1990). Ultrashort sleep strategies during sustained operations: the recuperative value of 80-, 50- and 20-min naps. In Shiftwork: health, sleep and performance (ed. G. Costa, G. Cesana, K, Kogi, and A. Wedderburn) Peter Lang, Frankfurt.

6

Time-zone transitions

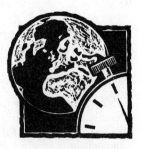

Since the Earth is spinning on its axis, for anybody standing on the Earth's surface, the sun rises in the east and sets in the west, and is at its highest point in the sky at noon by local time. However, these events must occur in the UK after they have taken place in countries to the east and before they have taken place in countries to the west. In order to resolve this problem, the world has been divided into 24 time-zones centred around Greenwich and separated by lines of longitude 15° apart. These time-zones determine the relationship between Greenwich Mean Time (GMT) and local time, those to the east of the UK being advanced and those to the west being delayed. Thus, at the same moment, it might be midday in the UK, but, by local time, 16:00 in Afghanistan, 21:00 in Japan, 07:00 in New York and 04:00 in Los Angeles. Thus, travelling to the east means you 'lose' time (in the sense that part of the day appears to have been lost), while travelling to the west means you 'gain' it (in the sense that you can relive some hours). This poses a problem when you travel to the antipodes, as you cross the international dateline, which is just to the east of New Zealand and separating Siberia and Alaska. At noon Monday on GMT, it will be midnight at the antipodes at the very end of Monday if you have travelled eastwards (12 hours ahead), but midnight at the very beginning of Monday if you have travelled westwards. This paradox was used by Jules Verne in his book, *Around the world in 80 days*.

For the seafarer or passenger on a cruise liner, the biological implications of time-zones are not very important. The rate of travel and of crossing time-zones is slow enough to be accommodated easily by the bodyclock. (As shown in Chapter 1, the bodyclock is a poor time-keeper and normally has to be adjusted each day by zeitgebers anyway). Sailing to New York, for example, entails putting the clock back 1–2 hours each day; in effect, you can stay up late, have a lie–in, and still be 'on schedule' by changing local time.

6.1 Jetlag

Problems arise when you cross several time-zones in a short space of time. Jet travellers suffer from a ragbag of symptoms, collectively known as 'jetlag'. The symptoms vary between individuals in details of their nature and severity, but include some or all of those shown in Table 6.1. Overall, they represent a general malaise or feeling of disorientation.

Table 6.1 Symptoms associated with the phenomenon of jetlag

Fatigue during the new daytime, and yet inability to sleep at night
Decreased mental performance, particularly if vigilance is required
Decreased physical performance, particularly in events needing stamina or precise
  movement
A loss of appetite, coupled with indigestion and even nausea
Increased irritability, headaches, mental confusion and disorientation

---

Sleep loss is of particular concern, since it causes decrements in mental performance (Chapter 3), and lowers mood states. The kind of difficulty depends upon the direction of flight. After eastward flights, it is getting to sleep that is more difficult; after ones to the west, it is staying asleep.

Only a few studies have looked specifically at sports performance after time-zone transitions (e.g. Shephard 1984; O'Connor and Morgan 1990; Reilly 1990). Studies on footballers indicate a poorer performance in the days immediately after the flight, though, as with field studies generally, a detailed explanation of the result is impossible due to insufficient data and the presence of other confounding influences (new surroundings and so on). Nevertheless, the effect is important for serious competition and agrees with results from closely controlled laboratory simulations of time-zone transitions. These simulations show that there is a loss of sleep and a general decline in motivation and physical and mental performance. In particular, the normal daytime peaks are blunted.

The problems arise because the bodyclock is slow to adjust to the new time-zone. This resistance to change is normally beneficial (Chapter 1), since it means that the bodyclock does not adjust inappropriately. For example, if we go to the cinema in the daytime, the clock does not adjust to the 'night', or if we raid the larder in the middle of the night the clock does not adjust to the 'day'. But this inertia of the clock, which is beneficial in these circumstances, is inappropriate after a time-zone transition. There will be a mismatch between body time and local time as illustrated for a subject who has just flown eight time-zones to the east (Table 6.2).

Table 6.2 Mismatch between local time and body time after a flight from UK to Hong Kong

New local time	Requirement	Body time	Desire
08:00	Waking	24:00	Going to sleep
16:00	Peak activity	08:00	Beginning to wake up
24:00	Retiring	16:00	Peak activity

When the circadian rhythms of body temperature, physical and mental performance are considered, then they correspond fully with this view (Wegmann and Klein 1985). Thus, in the example of an eastward flight across eight time-zones, minimum body temperature tends to fall at midday local time and the maximum body temperature at midnight. As a consequence of the links between temperature, sleep, and mental performance, sleep will be difficult to achieve and maintain at the new nighttime. The resulting fatigue will give rise to negative feelings, including irritability and headache. Mental and physical performance and mood will deteriorate, not only because they are taking place at times too far removed from the circadian peak, but also because the subjects will be unable to sleep properly (Chapter 3).

Other changes that are associated with a longhaul flight (Chapter 7) include:

1. a change of customs, including food;
2. the hassle of travel;
3. the loss of sleep due to the flight schedule;
4. anxiety due to the meeting in the new time-zone.

Do these other factors contribute to jetlag? To be sure, they do contribute to disturbing an individual, but changes (2) and (3) are essentially over within hours, whereas jetlag can last for five or more days. Additional reasons why the above factors are not a sufficient explanation of jetlag are:

1. The problems also arise when returning home.
2. The problems do not arise when flying a long way south, but without crossing many time-zones, e.g. from the UK to Sao Paulo or Johannesburg.
3. The problems do not depend much upon whether it is a night or day flight, i.e. the amount of sleep lost during the flight.
4. The problems depend far more upon time-zone changes than cultural changes. For example, jetlag is far worse when travelling from the UK to New Zealand than to Central Africa.
5. The problems can be reproduced in laboratory-based experiments. In this case, none of the other factors applies; the only change is in the local time.

These findings, particularly (5), and all other studies on circadian rhythms, confirm the view that jetlag is a function of the abnormal relationship between external and body time. Such problems will persist until the individual's rhythms resynchronize with the new time-zone.

6.2 Differences between flights and individuals

Accepting this desynchrony between body time and local time as the main cause of the problems, and knowing some of the properties of the body's timing system (Chapter 1), we can understand why jetlag is worse after an eastward flight and why some individuals are affected more than others.

Adjustment to a westward flight requires individuals to go to bed and wake up later, and for their bodyclock to delay; by contrast, adjustment to an eastward flight requires going to bed and rising earlier, and advancing the bodyclock. Going to bed earlier than is habitual is unlikely to be conducive to getting a full night's sleep. Not only are blood adrenaline and body temperature too high, but the individual has not been awake long enough to become tired. The resulting poor sleep is an inadequate preparation for the next full day, and the problem is exacerbated by the fact that by the time the body is ready to sleep the new local time indicates that it is time to get up for the next day! By contrast, after a westward flight, the increase in time spent awake before the new bedtime will tend to promote sleep and to offset the fact that it is being attempted when body temperature and adrenaline are rising. Thus, more sleep is obtained after a westward than an eastward flight, even though it still tends to finish too soon.

In addition, the bodyclock can delay more easily than advance, probably because its free-running period is greater than 24 h (Chapter 1). As a result, eastward flights, which require the clock to advance, are associated with a longer resynchronization time than are ones to the west but which entail crossing the same number of time-zones. Also, after a flight to the antipodes, where the time-shift is about 12 hours, adjustment is almost invariably by delay of the bodyclock. Indeed, this tendency for the bodyclock to delay rather than advance is so strong in some individuals that adjustment to an eastward flight across only nine time-zones (e.g. UK to Japan) is achieved not by an advance of body rhythms but rather by a 15-hour delay.

This last result stresses the differences between individuals when the process of adjustment is considered. Age is a disadvantage, in spite of the fact that individuals might be more experienced in flying and so more prepared to take advice to ameliorate jetlag. The increasing severity of jetlag with age probably occurs because older people are more set in their habits–particularly their sleep times and routines. Extremes, such as larks and owls (Chapter 1), are likely to respond differently to time-zone transitions (though there has been little systematic study of such subgroups). Larks, with a bodyclock that runs faster than average, would be predicted to have less difficulty with eastward flights, but more difficulty with those to the west. For owls, the westward flights should prove little problem but eastward ones are likely to pose considerable difficulty; it is likely that a substantial proportion of these individuals will adjust by a delay rather than an advance of their bodyclock.

6.3 Promoting adjustment in the new time-zone

It must be stated at the outset that many 'remedies' are little more than 'old wives' tales and that even some methods claiming scientific backing are poorly tested. Moreover, some methods that do work are not easy to implement for other reasons.

One approach is to tackle what many feel is the worst aspect of jetlag–the loss of sleep. Sleeping tablets and taking naps are considered in Chapter 5, and further consideration of their use by athletes is given in Chapter 7.

6.3.1 Short-acting hypnotics and naps

Getting to sleep and staying asleep are major problems. The use of short-acting hypnotics and the benzodiazepine group, in particular, has been useful in a military context (Nicholson 1984). In practice, it is not sending persons to sleep that is the problem but rather making sure that they are fully awake and alert when they are next on duty. This is because there may be problems due to the 'washout' time of the drug or of an active metabolite. For these reasons, when high levels of mental and physical performance are required, individuals should be very cautious about the use of sleeping tablets.

As an alternative, the use of naps or short sleeps, might be encouraged. As described previously (Chapter 5), naps can be taken at many times of the day and can serve as an aid to recuperation. They must not be too long, however, particularly if it is night on 'home-time'. This is because naps that are too long will make you less likely to sleep at the new nighttime, and sleeps taken at night on home-time are likely to prevent adjustment of the bodyclock.

Since the problems of jetlag stem from a desynchronization between local and body time, methods of promoting the adjustment of the bodyclock have been used. This becomes a matter of strengthening zeitgebers in the new time-zone.

6.3.2 Melatonin capsules

In normal circumstances, melatonin secretion from the pineal gland is a very reliable marker of the bodyclock and is secreted into the bloodstream between about 21:00 and 07:00. It can be regarded as a 'dark pulse' or 'internal zeitgeber'. Several studies have shown that melatonin capsules taken in the evening by local time in the new time-zone reduce the symptoms of 'jetlag' (Arendt *et al.* 1987). This is an important finding, but there are some caveats:

1. Jetlag, as defined in these studies, has concentrated on subjective symptoms; we do not know if there would also be improvements in mental and physical performance, and in motivation to train hard, or even if there would be further decrements.

2. It is not clear if melatonin produces its effect by promoting adjustment of the bodyclock or by some other means (e.g. increasing a sense of well-being or the ability to sleep). Recent work suggests that melatonin should adjust the bodyclock, but this requires the careful timing of ingestion, according to whether you wish to advance or delay the clock (Lewy *et al.* 1992). Thus, melatonin taken in the evening (on body time) will advance the bodyclock, and when taken in the morning will delay it.
3. Melatonin is only just becoming commercially available and the results from many clinical trials are still awaited.

In summary, more information is required before melatonin can be recommended.

6.3.3 The timing and composition of meals

It has been argued that high-protein breakfasts promotes alertness and that high-carbohydrate evening meals promote sleep (Graeber *et al.* 1981). The theoretical grounds for this include the effects upon plasma amino acids that such meals have and, thence, the uptake of amino acids into the brain, their incorporation into neurotransmitters, and the release of the neurotransmitters. High-protein meals undoubtedly raise plasma tyrosine, but it is less clear whether this promotes the release of catecholamines by the activating systems of the brain, and so promotes alertness. Similarly, high-carbohydrate meals promote the concentration of plasma tryptophan, but it is also uncertain whether this stimulates the raphe nucleus and sleep (Leathwood 1989). The method was promoted in the USA (under the title 'President Reagan's anti-jetlag diet'), but the scientific tests of the efficacy of the diet are few and poorly designed.

Even so, a variant of this proposal has been marketed. It consists of two types of pills, one to be taken in the morning and the other in the evening. Each pill is a mixture of substances, the morning-pill containing tyrosine and the evening pill, tryptophan. The literature accompanying the medication does not enable a judgement to be made on the scientific evaluation of these preparations.

6.3.4 Bright-light exposure and physical activity

Bright light (i.e., of an intensity found naturally but not normally indoors) appears to be a potent zeitgeber in humans and can adjust the bodyclock. The timing of exposure to it is crucially important (Czeisler *et al.* 1989; Minors *et al.* 1991) and is the opposite of that for melatonin ingestion; thus, bright light in the morning (05:00–11:00) on body time advances the clock, and bright light in the evening (21:00–03:00) on body time delays it. As a supplement to this treatment, there are also times when light should be avoided (those times which produce a shift of the body clock in a direction opposite to that desired). In addition, if melatonin has its effect by adjusting the bodyclock (see above), then at such times as light is avoided it would also be appropriate for melatonin (the 'dark pulse') to be taken. Table 6.3 gives times when light should be sought or avoided after different time-zone transitions.

Table 6.3 The use of bright light to adjust the bodyclock after time-zone transitions

	Bad local times for exposure to bright light	Good local times for exposure to bright light
Time zones to the west		
4 hours	01:00–07:00*	17:00–23:00†
8 hours	21:00–03:00*	13:00–19:00†
12 hours	17:00–23:00*	09:00–15:00†
Time zones to the east		
4 hours	01:00–07:00†	09:00–15:00*
8 hours	05:00–11:00†	13:00–19:00*
12 hours	Treat this as 12 hours to the west	

* Will advance the bodyclock
† Will delay the bodyclock

Even though 'bright light' is of an intensity normally not achieved in domestic or interior lighting, light boxes and visors are now available commerically that produce a light source of sufficient intensity. In particular, light visors might prove a useful addition to one's luggage.

Since outdoor lighting is the obvious choice, it would therefore be natural to consider training outdoors, e.g. a brisk walk, swim, or game of tennis, when light is required, and to relax indoors when it should be avoided. This raises the question whether physical exercise and inactivity can somehow substitute for light and dark, respectively. Current data are not yet convincing, though this would be the result if humans were like hamsters in this regard (Mrosovsky *et al.* 1989). In practice, it would therefore seem that combing exposure to bright light with exercise, while combining dim light with relaxation, would seem advisable to those wanting to adjust to the new time-zone.

6.4. 'When in Rome . . .'

To a large extent, the best advice is to adjust as fully as possible to the lifestyle and habits in the new time-zone. This is not always the case in the first day or so after the flight. Consider, first, a westward flight through eight time-zones. To delay the bodyclock, bright light is needed at 21:00–03:00 body time and should be avoided at 05:00–11:00. By the new local time, this becomes equal to 13:00–19:00 for bright light and 21:00–03:00 for dim light (see Table 6.3). It can be seen that natural daylight and night would provide this. Consider, by contrast, a flight to the east through eight times zones. In this instance, light is required at 05:00–11:00 body time (13:00–19:00 local time) and should be avoided at 21:00–03:00 body time (05:00–11:00 local time). Thus, for the first day or so, morning light would be unhelpful and tend to make the body clock adjust in the wrong direction (though light in the afternoon and evening is appropriate).

Just as with the time of ingestion of melatonin (see above), the timing of exposure to bright light is therefore critical on the first days after the flight. After a couple of days, when adjustment will be partial, it is then advisable to adjust the timing of light exposure towards that of the local inhabitants, to enable your habits to become fully synchronized with theirs.

6.5 Overview

For the traveller, the days immediately after a longhaul flight can be dispiriting, with lack of motivation, poor sleep, and decreased mental and physical performance. Again, understanding the cause can be some consolation psychologically, and the aim must be to promote adjustment to the new time-zone as quickly as possible. These issues are further addressed in the context of the travelling athlete in the next chapter.

Further reading

Graeber, R. C. (1989). Jet-lag and sleep disruption. In *Principles and practice of sleep medicine* (ed. M. J. Kryger, T. Roth, and W. C. Dement), pp. 324–31. Saunders, Philadelphia.

Winget, C. M., DeRoshia C. W., Markley, C. L., and Holley, D. C. (1984). A review of human physiological and performance changes associated with desynchronosis of biological rhythms. *Aviat. Space Environ. Med.*, **55**, 1085–96.

References

Arendt, J., Aldhous, M., English, J., Marks, V., and Folkard, S. (1987). Some effects of jet-lag and their alleviation by melatonin. *Ergonomics*, **30**, 1379–93

Czeisler, C., Kronauer, R., and Allan, J. (1989). Bright light induction of strong (type 0) resetting of the human circadian pacemaker. *Science*, **244**, 1328–333.

Graeber, R., Sing, H., and Cuthbert, B. (1981). The impact of transmeridian flight on deploying soliders. In *Biological rhythms, sleep and shift work* (ed. L. Johnson, D. Tepas, and W. Colquhoun), pp.513–37, MTP Press, Lancaster.

Leathwood, P. (1989). Circadian rhythms of plasma amino acids, brain neurotransmitters and behaviour. In *Biological rhythms in clinical practice* (ed. J. Arendt, D. Minors, and J. Waterhouse), pp.136–59. Wright, Bristol.

Lewy, A., Ahmed, S., Lathan Jackson, J., and Sack, R. (1992). Melatonin shifts human circadian rhythms according to a phase-response curve. *Chronobiol. Int.*, **9**, 380–92.

Minors, D., Waterhouse, J., and Wirz-Justice, A. (1991). A human phase-response curve to light. *Neurosci. Lett.*, **133**, 36–40.

Mrosovsky, N., Reebs, S., Honrado, G., and Salmon, P. (1989). Behavioural entrainment of circadian rhythms. *Experientia*, **45**, 696–702.

Nicholson, A. (1984). Long periods of work and sleep. *Ergonomics*, **27**, 629–30.

O'Connor, P. and Morgan, W. (1990). Athletic performance following rapid traversal of multiple time zones. *Sports Med.*, **10**, 20–30.

Reilly, T. (1990). Human circadan rhythms and exercise. *Crit Rev. Biomed. Eng.*, **8**, 165–80.

Shephard, R. (1984). Sleep, biorhythms and human performance. *Sports Med.*, **1**, 11–37.

Wegmann, H. and Klein, K. (1985). Jet-lag and aircrew scheduling. In *Hours of work* (ed. S. Folkard and T. Monk), pp.263–76. Wiley, Chichester.

Further information on light visors can be obtained in the UK from: Outside In (Cambridge) Ltd., Unit 3, Scotland Road Estate, Dry Drayton, Cambridge, CB3 8AT, England, UK. The address to write to in the USA is: Bio-Brite Inc., 7315 Wisconsin Avenue, Suite 1300 W, Bethesda, MD 20814–3202, USA.

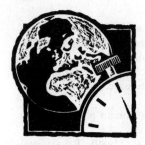

7
The travelling athlete

7.1 Introduction

Competitive sport is now recognized on a global scale and people at many levels, from the Olympic Games athlete to the recreational runner, have the opportunity of competing abroad. Travelling to strange places for purposes of competing in sport seems highly alluring. In reality, this foreign travel makes great demands on team-managers, athletes, and coaches, whether they are planning trips abroad for a single competition or a prolonged tour. Whatever country is the destination, a vast surveillance exercise is called for to glean information about the culture and customs of the host country, the immunization necessary, climatic factors including temperature, seasonal variations in climate, altitude, and so on.

Guidelines are necessary for dealing with changes in temperature (heat and cold), pressure (altitude), cuisine (nutrition), and travel. Our concern here is with the problems encountered by athletes as a result of crossing time-zones, which are very different in nature from the 'travel-fatigue' experienced after flying North or South or after long journeys in cars or buses. Regular walks on the plane, some stretching, and isometrics will all help to minimize this form of fatigue during flights. At the end of the journey, a refreshing shower or a good night's sleep will be totally restorative. This is not the case after quickly crossing time-zones, either coast to coast in Australia or North America, across continental Europe or Asia, or transoceanic flights.

The physiological disturbances associated with rapid time-zone transitions have been described in Chapter 6. Their relevance to, and effects, on athletes' performances are explained in this chapter. The suitability of various procedures for coping with 'jetlag' are also examined.

7.2 Jetlag

The feelings of disorientation encountered as a result of crossing time-zones are known as jetlag. The physiological basis for their occurrence was presented in Chapter 6. Symptoms include fatigue and general tiredness, inability to sleep at night, loss of concentration, loss of drive, headaches, and general malaise. Sufferers may have bizarre lapses in mental attention and unusual errors in short-term memory. These problems are a consequence of disrupting the body's normal rhythms as a result of rapid transitions across multiple time-zones. Such desynchronization of rhythms is similar in principle to that which occurs in nocturnal shiftwork employees following their transfer to night-shifts. A difference is that travellers across time-zones must fit in with all aspects of local time in the new environment. This is especially important in athletes who generally want to maintain their training habit or continue a systematic build-up for a forthcoming contest.

7.3 Circadian desynchronization

Following a journey across multiple time-zones, the body's rhythms at first retain the characteristics of their point of departure. The new environment soon forces new influences on these cycles, the main factors being the time of sunrise and onset of darkness. The body attempts to adjust to this new context, but some functions such as core temperature are relatively sluggish in doing so. As a rough guide, it can take up to one day for each time-zone crossed for body temperature to adapt completely. The individual may have difficulty in sleeping for a few days, but activity and social contact during the day help to accelerate the adaptation of the arousal rhythm. Thus, arousal adjusts more quickly than does body temperature to the new time-zone. Until the whole spectrum of biological rhythms adjusts to the new local time, thereby becoming resynchronized, the performance of exercise may be below par. An example is travel between the UK and Australia. The phase of the oral-temperature curve is shifted to the left when going eastwards (Fig. 7.1*a*) and to the right (Fig. 7.1*b*) on the return flight. In both directions, there was a brief stopover in Singapore.

Allowing for individual differences, the severity of jetlag is affected by a variety of factors. In general, the greater the number of time-zones crossed, the more difficult it is to cope. A two-hour phase shift may have marginal significance but a three-hour shift (e.g. British or Irish teams travelling to play European football matches in Russia or the Middle East, or a Californian sports team travelling to play on the east coast of the U S A) will entail desynchronisation to a substantial degree. In such cases, the flight times – time of departure and time of arrival – may determine how severe are the symptoms of jetlag.

The severity of symptoms may be worse 2–3 days after arrival than on the day immediately following disembarkation. Symptoms then gradually abate, but can still be acute at particular times of day. There will be a window of time during the day when the period of high arousal associated with the time-zone just left overlaps with peak arousal for the new local time. This window may be predicted in advance and should be used to time training practices in the first few days at destination. Our observations on footballers travelling eastwards from Britain to Oceania (Australia, New Zealand, and Papua New

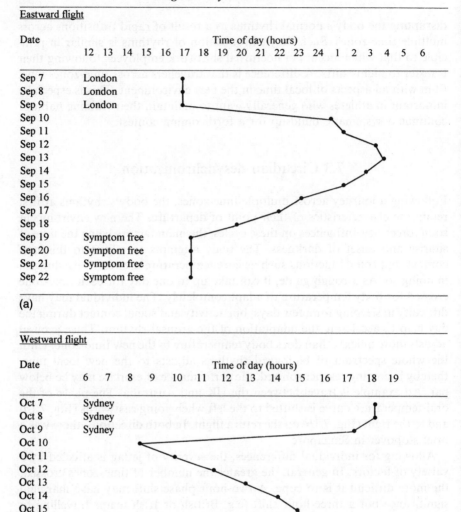

(a)

(b)

Fig. 7.1 Peak time of day is plotted for oral temperature after an eastward journey to Australia from the UK (top) and after the return home (bottom). The time shown is local time. The graph shows that symptoms of jetlag disappeared about the time that body temperature returned to its normal rhythm.

Guinea) indicate that morning training sessions (after 11:00) suit players best over the first few days (Reilly and Mellor 1988). Such a practice has also proved successful for cross-country runners after travelling from Britain to compete in Australia and New Zealand. This advice may not apply to athletes travelling westwards, for example, Australians travelling to compete in Europe.

The British Rugby League players who travelled to Australia showed a disturbance in their circadian rhythm in grip strength. By the fourth day, strength values in the evening were higher than the morning scores (Table 7.1). It took 2–3 more days for the normal circadian rhythm to restore itself.

Table 7.1 Grip strength (N) for 4 days after the day of arrival in Sydney from London. (Mean ± SD.)

Day	Morning	Evening
1	484.1 ± 42.4	476.2 ± 44.4
2	486.1 ± 44.4	478.2 ± 46.3
3	484.1 ± 43.4	487.1 ± 45.4
4	481.2 ± 42.2	496.9 ± 47.3 7

Effects of jetlag may be evident in football players travelling within one country. An analysis of American football results indicated that teams travelling from west to central or eastern zones were adversely affected, except when matches were played at night. West Coast teams playing at home in the evening were at an advantage (Jehue *et al.* 1993). When going eastwards, the mean performance is depressed more and the peak performance declines more dramatically than is the case when travelling westwards. Altering training times for a few days prior to travel to reflect the time of competition in another time-zone is known to be beneficial (Jehue *et al.* 1993). Similar trends are likely to prevail in Australian Rules football teams travelling across Australia, or in European soccer teams travelling across time-zones for competitive matches.

The direction of travel affects the severity of jetlag. As explained in Chapters 1 and 6, it is easier to cope with flying in a westward direction compared to flying eastwards. In flying westwards, the normal cycle is temporarily lengthened and body rhythms can extend in line with their natural freerunning period of about 25 hours and thus catch up. Observations on athletes travelling to Korea (9 hours in advance of British Summer Time) and Malaysia (7 hours in advance of British Summer Time) are that periods of 9 and 6 days, respectively, may be inadequate for jetlag symptoms to disappear. In contrast, readaptation is more rapid on returning to Britain. When time-zone shifts approach near to maximal values – the maximum is a 12-hour change – there may be little difference between eastward and westward travel but adjustment of the bodyclock is nearly always by delay.

The period of time necessary to adjust to the timing of a new country's environmental cycles may depend on the time of day at which competitions are scheduled. O'Connor *et al* (1991) recorded changes that seemed to show improved performances for swimmers following a westward flight across four time-zones. These changes included an improved mood and a decreased rating of perceived exertion. The swimmers were tested at 13:00 local time on arrival: this time would correspond to early evening according to the swimmers' unadjusted bodyclock, and is the time of day at which performance is normally at its best.

Young individuals have a better tolerance to desynchronization of rhythms due to a better regulation of biological clocks. Older individuals tend to suffer more from jetlag than do younger people. Physical fitness also seems to play a role, with physically active subjects demonstrating higher amplitudes in existing rhythms than age-matched controls – a difference indicative of superior regulation. The higher amplitude of the rhythms in fit individuals means that the rhythms are more stable and resistant to change. The better tolerance of athletes travelling across time-zones may be due to the zeitgeber qualities of the exercise they perform on arrival in this new time-zone.

Both men and women suffer symptoms of jetlag although the severity of symptoms may be related to the menstrual-cycle phase. Disruptions of the menstrual cycle in female travellers have been linked to disturbances in melatonin secretion. Higher melatonin levels in the Scandinavian winter compared with summer values have an inhibiting effect on luteinizing hormone. As a consequence, ovulation may not occur during that cycle (Harma *et al.* 1994). It is not known to what extent the menstrual disturbances accompanying travelling across multiple time-zones, in themselves, alter the performances or exercise capabilities of female athletes.

7.4 Reducing jetlag in athletes

On lengthy journeys, it is unlikely that any manoeuvres will completely eliminate jetlag, but careful planning can attenuate the symptoms. In the week before departure, it may be possible to adjust the time of arising and going to bed, the adjustment depending on the direction of flight. A change of more than 2 hours is likely to be unproductive since this would interfere with the pattern of social and domestic engagements during the day. Besides, the major synchronizer of human circadian rhythms – natural daylight – remains unaltered. In practice, few travellers have the opportunity or the motivation to change their sleeping times before going overseas.

The evidence from simply adjusting the time of retiring to sleep (Reilly and Maskell 1989) is as follows:

1. Shifting the sleep – wake cycle does alter rhythms in accord with the direction of the shift but only partly.
2. However, motor performance is compromized during the course of such adaptive changes, with both the mean and amplitude being depressed.
3. Caution is advocated in manipulating the sleep – wakefulness rhythm prior to travelling to compete abroad.

Once flight-times are known, a routine on the plane may be planned. In daytime flights, it will be necessary to stay awake, keep mentally active, and perhaps watch the in-flight movie. On long-haul flights with travelling during the night, it will be necessary to get some sleep on the plane. The timing of this should be decided in advance so that some on-board meals can be missed. Transit or transfer episodes en route should be taken into consideration.

It is a good strategy to set one's watch to local time at the next point of landing, once on board the plane: in a single-haul flight, this would be the local time of the country of destination. The important thing is that the traveller mentally tunes in to the new local time straightaway and adjusts behaviour accordingly.

To compensate for the dry air during flight, copious rehydration is advised. Fruit juices are best, while fizzy drinks should be avoided. Alcohol should not be taken, since it acts as a diuretic causing loss of fluid, and also affects the normal circadian rhythm in renal function. Caffeine in coffee also stimulates water loss, and its arousal effect on the central nervous system (CNS) means that it should not be taken if sleep is desired. One suggestion is that the last meal prior to the time allotted for sleep should be high in carbohydrates and low in protein in order to induce drowsiness. This is because carbohydrates provide the amino-acid substrates for serotonin, a neurotransmitter which regulates sleep (Chapter 6). Caffeine and a low-carbohydrate high-protein breakfast would help raise the level of arousal and prevent a relapse into sleep.

Athletes may feel stiff or cramped because of their restrained posture during flight. They can perform isometric exercises for arms, trunk, or legs, while remaining in their seats. It is still better, however, to walk often down the aisle of the plane, and occasionally to do flexibility or stretching exercises at the back of the plane. This will also remind the athlete that the primary purpose of the trip is for sport and not tourism.

British sports teams travelling to Australia have used sleeping pills to induce sleep while on board. Military aircraft pilots flying from Britain to the Falkland Islands have also used minor tranquillizers (temazepam) to get to sleep so as to be refreshed for immediate activities, or for taking courage for the return journey. Although drugs, such as benzodiazepines, are effective in getting people to sleep, they do not guarantee a prolonged period asleep. Besides, they have not been satisfactorily tested for subsequent residual effects on motor performance, such as sports skills. They may be counter-productive if given at the incorrect time. A prolonged sleep at the time an individual feels drowsy (presumably when he or she would have been asleep in the time-zone departed from) simply anchors the rhythms at their former phases and so resists the adjustment to the new time-zone.

7.5 Arrival at destinations

On reaching the country of destination, a key factor is how well the athlete fits in immediately with the phase characteristics of the new environment. Athletes should already have worked out the local time for their disembarkation. There may be other environmental factors to consider, such as heat, humidity, or even altitude. The visiting team may even have to experience an entirely contrasting season, e.g. as when European teams travel to Australia and New Zealand, or to Argentina, Brazil, or Uruguay.

Having travelled westwards, players may be allowed to go to bed early. The early onset of sleep will be more likely than after an eastward flight. A light training session on the evening of arrival can help instill local cues into the rhythms. There is also some evidence that exercise speeds up the adaptation to a new time-zone.

Exercise, itself, provides a good signal for adjustment of the biological clock to the new time-zone. The observations in Figure 7.2 are on a Premier League football team returning to England from Japan. Rather than go to bed, the players went straight from the airport to the team's training ground, having arrived at midday. Training was light in intensity and players returned home in the late afternoon with advice on when to retire to sleep. Their jetlag problems were clearly reduced compared with other trips when their behaviour was uncontrolled.

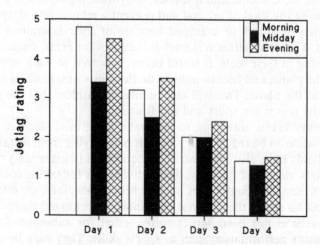

Fig. 7.2 Jetlag symptoms at three times of the day on professional soccer players on return from a Far-East tournament.

For the first few days in the new time-zone, training sessions should not be all-out efforts. Skills requiring fine coordination are likely to be impaired and this may lead to accidents or injuries if, for example, games players conduct sessions with the ball too strenuously. When a series of tournament engagements is scheduled, it is useful to have at least one friendly match during the initial period, that is, before the end of the first week in the overseas country.

During this period of adaptation, a few caveats are noted. Alcohol taken late in the evening is likely to disrupt sleep and so is not advised. The alternation of feasting and fasting recommended for commercial travellers in the USA. (with the intention of altering substrate for neurotransmitter substances) is unlikely to gain acceptance among runners, cyclists, or footballers. Nevertheless, they could benefit from biasing the macronutrients in their evening meal largely towards carbohydrates. These would include vegetables with a choice of chipped, roast, or baked potatoes, pasta dishes, rice, and bread. These should also include sufficient fibre to safeguard against constipation.

In the early days in the new country, athletes should be discouraged from taking long naps. A nap at the time they would have been asleep had they stayed at home will make subsequent sleep more difficult and retard adjustment of the biological clock to the new regimen. Exposure to bright light, preferably natural daylight, is a useful antidote to drowsiness in such circumstances and also has phase-shifting effects (see Chapter 6 for details).

Taking drugs can alter the biological clock, but their effects depend on the time they are taken. Caffeine (in coffee) and theophylline (in tea) are CNS stimulants. If taken in the evening, they help in recovery after flying eastwards, and if taken in the afternoon, after flying westwards.

The minor tranquillizers, the benzodiazepines, affect neurotransmitters that have a role in the arousal curve. These include serotonin, noradrenaline, acetylcholine, and gamma-aminobutyric acid (GABA). As already indicated, they are effective in inducing sleep, but not necessarily good in ensuring the state of sleep. Also, hangover effects cannot be excluded, even in some so-called short-acting hypnotics.

Administration of melatonin, which is a pineal gland hormone, has shown good results in treating Scandinavian patients suffering depression in the winter. This clinical condition is known as seasonal affective disorder (SAD) and seems to be rare among athletes. The lack of stimulus from natural light, which suppresses melatonin secretion by the pineal gland, is a recognized cause of SAD. Prolonged exposure to bright artificial light has also proved effective in these patients. Oral ingestion of melatonin tablets on a trip from Britain to Australia (Arendt *et al.* 1987) showed that subjects experienced:

(1) a reduction in jetlag symptoms;
(2) improvements in sleep quality;
(3) a faster readjustment of cortisol and melatonin rhythms.

These findings received further support from results of a simulated eastward flight across nine time-zones. However, toxic side-effects of this substance cannot be discounted, and it is not yet readily available in tablet form. Its effects on athletic performance are unknown.

There is also a suggestion that the amino acid 'tryptophan' is helpful in coping with jetlag (Chapter 6). It is a precursor of the sleep hormones, but there is no evidence that it improves the quality of sleep. It also received bad publicity in the early 1990s, when impurities were found in commercially available products, and its use is no longer recommended.

It is more effective to use bright light or behavioural measures to resynchronize circadian rhythms. Natural daylight and bright artificial light help to increase or maintain arousal, and also help the endogenous rhythms to get into phase with the local environment. For athletes, exercise is a powerful resynchronizor, as mentioned already. It stimulates catecholamines and alertness. It is recommended, even on the day of arrival, except late in the evening local time. Exercise of a light-to-moderate intensity is adequate for stimulating the resynchronization of rhythmic characteristics, since exercise that is too strenuous may disrupt rather than promote sleep.

A system of self-monitoring of jetlag and sleep quality (Fig. 7.3) can provide great information about the time taken to adjust to the new time-zone. This allows the coach to monitor a travelling squad, as well as to educate the athletes about the symptoms. The system has been used by British athletes at their Olympic training camp in Florida. Observations have confirmed that it generally takes 4–6 days to be completely clear of jetlag following a flight across the Atlantic, while sleep is satisfactory in most athletes after 3 nights.

7.6 Overview and recommendations

If it is possible to do so, flights should be scheduled so that athletes arrive well in advance of competition. One day for each time-zone crossed leaves a margin of safety, even when travelling eastwards. The time for adaptation may be shortened by exploiting the external factors that reset biological clocks, such as rest/exercise, darkness/light, meals, and social influences. The key is to tune in straight away to the external influences of the new environment.

It may be beneficial to shop around to find the most convenient travel schedules. Consider a departure from a regional airport, if appropriate, and also alternative carriers. The routines prior to departure, on the plane, and after arrival can be planned once the itinerary is established. In consequence, coping with jetlag will not be the trial-and-error affair it might otherwise be.

Instructions to athlete
Please estimate the time at which you go to sleep and the time at which you awake.
Place a mark on the sleep–quality scale to describe how well you slept. Please also
make a note of the time and length of any naps that you have (including during the
flight). A space for other notes is on the back page.

Name ....   Date of birth ....

Date of flight from England ....   Time of departure ....

Date of arrival ....   Time of arrival ....

Day 1 in USA

Morning (time   )   Midday (time   )

1--2--3--4--5--6--7--8--9--10   1--2--3--4--5--6--7--8--9--10
↑   ↑   ↑   ↑
Normal   Strongest jet   Normal   Strongest jet
                 lag imaginable   lag imaginable

Right grip   Right grip

Left grip   Left grip

Oral temperature   Oral temperature

Evening (time   )   Night (time   )

1--2--3--4--5--6--7--8--9--10   1--2--3--4--5--6--7--8--9--10
↑   ↑   ↑   ↑
Normal   Strongest jet   Normal   Strongest jet
                 lag imaginable   lag imaginable

Right grip   Right grip

Left grip   Left grip

Oral temperature   Oral temperature

Fig. 7.3 Example of a scale for monitoring the effects of jetlag on athletes
travelling to the USA. Data were collected also on grip strength and oral
temperature at four times a day.

By preparing for time-zone transitions and the disturbances they impose on the body's rhythms, the severity of jetlag symptoms can be reduced. There has been little success in attempting to predict good and poor adaptors to long-haul flights. Athletes are generally better than nonathletes in coping with jetlag and they tend not to suffer as much. The fact that an individual escapes lightly from symptoms on one occasion is no guarantee that he or she will do so again on the next visit. The disturbances in mental performance and cognitive functions have consequences not only for sports performers, but also for the management and medical staff travelling with the team, who by no means have immunity against jetlag. An awareness of the dynamic biological adjustments that the body is making means that the adverse effects and discomfort associated with jetlag can be countered to some degree.

Further reading

de Looy, A. E., Minors, D. S., Waterhouse, J., Reilly T., and Tunstall-Pedoe, D. (1988). *The coach's guide to competing abroad.* National Coaching Foundation, Leeds.

Minors, D. S., and Waterhouse, J. M. (1981). *Circadian rhythms and the human.* Wright, Bristol.

Minors, D. S., Waterhouse, J. M., and Smith, L. R. (1993). The body clock: jet-lag, physical and psychological rhythms. In: *Intermittent high intensity exercise: preparation, stresses and damage limitation* (ed. D.A.D. Macleod, R. J. Maughan, C. Williams, G. R. Madeley, J. C. M. Sharp, and R. W. Nutton, pp. 375–90. Spon, London.

Reilly, T. (1987). Circadian rhythms and exercise. In: *Exercise, benefits, limits and adaptations* (ed. D. Macleod, R. J. Maughan, M. Nimmo, T. Reilly, and C. Williams, pp. 346–6 London.

US Olympic Committee. (1988). *From the US to Seoul.* US Olympic Committee, Colorado Springs.

References

Arendt, J., Aldhous, M., English, J., Marks, J., Arendt, J. H., Marks, M., and Folkard, S. (1987). Some effects of jet-lag and their alteration by melatonin. *Ergonomics,* **30**, 1379–94.

Harma, M., Laitinen, J., Partinen, M., and Savanto, S. (1994). The effect of four-day round trip flights over 10 time zones on the circadian variation of salivary melatonin and cortisol in airline flight attendants. *Ergonomics,* **37**, 1479–89.

Jehue, R., Street, D., and Huizenga, R. (1993). Effect of time zone and game time changes in team performance: National Football League. Med. Sci. Sports Exerc., **25**, 127–31.

O'Connor, P. T., Morgan, W. P., Koltyn, K. F., Raglin, J. S., Turner, J. G., and

Kalin, N. H. (1991). Air travel across four time zones in college swimmers. *J. App. Physiol.*, **70**, 756–63.

Reilly, T. and Maskell, P. (1989). Effects of altering the sleep–wake cycle on human circadian rhythms and motor performance. In Proceedings First IOC Congress on Sports Sciences (Colorado Springs), pp. 106–107.

Reilly, T. and Mellor, S. (1988). Jet-lag in student Rugby League players following a near maximal time-zone shift. In *Science and football* (ed. T. Reilly, A. Lees, K. Davids, and W. J. Murphy, pp. 249–56. Spon, London.

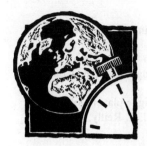

8
Shiftwork

8.1 Introduction

Like transmeridian travel, participation in shiftwork can disrupt human circadian rhythms. It should be noted that crossing time-zones and working shifts are not chronobiologically identical. When multiple time-zones are crossed, a person is normally exposed to all the zeitgebers of the new environment, whereas during rotating shiftwork that includes nightwork, any change in the phasing of a person's rhythms has occurred while being exposed to some zeitgebers still associated with a diurnal existence (e.g. the light–dark cycle). A consideration of shiftwork is further complicated by the fact that the rhythm disturbances may not be isolated events, as in trans-meridian travel, but can be frequent, occurring every time a shift may rotate. In this chapter, shiftwork schedules and their effects on the human are discussed. The influence of working unusual hours on performance and leisure pursuits are given special attention. Solutions to the problem of shiftwork are also examined through the application of chronobiological theory.

8.2 The importance of shiftwork

Many occupations, due to their social or economic importance need to operate 24 hours per day. This phenomenon is not new. Although many preindustrial peasants in Britain enjoyed a four-day working week (Monday was devoted to boxing and blood sports), with most work scheduled within the hours of daylight, it was still necessary for some people to work at night. Deliveries in and around ancient Rome were made only at night in order to alleviate traffic congestion (Scherrer 1981). 'Our daily bread' has been baked at night since biblical times or before. Today, the rate of participation in shiftwork is 10–25 per cent of all those employed. Rates may be higher than this in specific populations, such as British male manual workers (34.3 per cent, Young 1982) and Americans employed in parttime work (47 per cent).

Although in the last 25 years, the number of hours worked per week has been reduced, the number of shiftworkers in the European Union has doubled over the same period (Roberts and Chambers 1985). This suggests that most people now have a greater amount of leisure-time, but that recreational pursuits are still scheduled for many at unsociable or impractical times of day.

Most people working in modern manufacturing industries regard shiftwork as occupational bouts, the start and finish times of which may be periodically changed 'around the clock', including the hours of darkness. Many other individuals would consider that they are shiftworkers, even though they do not work through all the nocturnal hours or in such a structured, rotating schedule. For example, postal and milk-delivery workers are on permanent early morning-shifts. Junior doctors may be 'on call' for over 50 hours with only short periods of sleep. Permanent nightworkers are often referred to as shiftworkers, even though their work-periods do not 'shift' at all to different times of the day. Such workers, however, often revert to a diurnal existence on their days off. As there are so many shiftwork schedules and because only a slight deviation from the 'normal' diurnal working period may result in problems for the worker, this chapter uses the broad definition provided by Monk and Folkard (1992). Shiftwork is therefore 'any regularly taken employment outside the day working window, defined arbitrarily as the hours between 07:00 and 18:00'.

8.3 The problems of shiftwork

The accurate description of problems associated with shiftwork is, in itself, a problem. Employers argue that shiftwork is necessary and shiftworkers are adequately compensated financially for any inconvenience that is incurred. Trade unions usually disagree and maintain that the disadvantages of shiftwork far outweigh the economic advantages. Unfortunately, these dichotomous views restrict the chronobiologist in carrying out shiftwork studies. Employers are worried that an experiment will distract the workers from performing their occupational tasks, whereas employees are concerned that any research is not for their own benefit, but that they are being scrutinized by employer-recruited spies. Both parties are worried that the results of an experiment will lead to interventions that compromise their interests. The main methodological problem when researching shiftwork is the measurement of sufficient aspects of 'tolerance' both quickly and accurately. Comparisons between shiftworkers and the general population are complicated by the fact that a significant number of people find shiftwork so difficult that it makes them leave their job. This means that the difficulties of shiftworkers may be underestimated if these 'drop-outs' are not examined. Despite these political and methodological constraints, researchers have been able to record reliably three main sources of shiftwork 'strain' (Monk and Folkard 1992). These are strain from circadian rhythm alterations, strain from sleep problems, and social and domestic strain. The shiftworking athlete may experience the added strain of disruption to leisure and sports interests.

8.3.1 Circadian rhythms and shiftwork

Rectal temperature has been measured continuously before, during, and after a bout of nightwork (Fig. 8.1). The acrophase of the body-temperature rhythm gradually shifts from about 19:00 on daywork to about 24:00 after 3 weeks of night-shifts (Knauth *et al.* 1978). Adjustment of the biological clock, however, cannot be considered to be complete at this time since the phase-change of the body-temperature rhythm is still not the same as the phase-change of the workshift. This phenomenon is believed to occur even when permanent nightshifts are worked, since workers are exposed to zeitgebers associated with a diurnal routine on their days off. When the rectal-temperature rhythm is 'unmasked' by correcting for the influences of sleep and activity, the adjustment of the endogenous component to nightwork is even less than that shown in Fig. 8.1. Not all rhythms are slow to adjust to nightwork. Heart rate and blood pressure, for example, entrain completely to nightwork during the first few days that the shift is worked (Baumgart *et al.* 1989). This suggests that, during shiftwork, the phase relationships between endogenous and exogenous rhythms will be different from those found under nychthemeral conditions. It is this 'internal dissociation' between different circadian rhythms that is thought to exacerbate the detrimental effects of shiftwork.

8.3.2 Shiftwork and sleep

Shiftworkers obtain less sleep than the 7.5–8.0 h reported by dayworkers. The quality of sleep (indicated by sleep stages) is also different during shiftwork, especially when sleep is attempted in the presence of noise. The reasons for the shiftworker's sleep deprivation are related to the sources of strain identified in the previous and following sections – disturbances in circadian rhythms and external social factors. First, the slow adjustment of the biological clock to nightwork means that the worker will be attempting to sleep when the bodyclock is signalling wakefulness. Second, diurnal sleepers are more exposed to disturbances and noise, both within the house and in the immediate surroundings. Noise is a huge problem for the daytime-sleeping shiftworker. Even when noise originating from within the house is adequately controlled, noise can emanate from children playing in the street, traffic, domestic services, or spectators at a nearby sports stadium. Although a single bout of slightly reduced sleep does not adversely affect exercise performance, the chronic sleep deprivation found in shiftworkers may decrease their ability to perform exercise.

8.3.3 Shiftwork and society

Homo sapiens is a diurnal creature. Consequently, 'normal' society expects people to work between 08:00 and 18:00 and to fulfil other roles outside these times. Abnormal hours of work engage with the timetables of neither other organizations or other citizens. The citizens most obviously affected by shiftwork, other than the shiftworkers themselves, are those in the family. Over 50 per cent of shiftworkers' partners are fairly or very unhappy about their spouses' hours of work (Smith and Folkard 1993). About 60–70% of

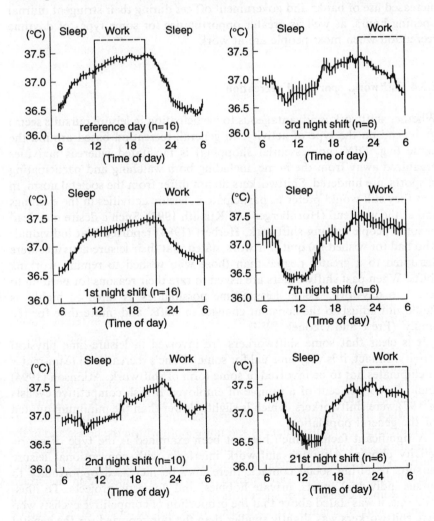

Fig. 8.1 Entrainment of the circadian rhythm in body temperature to a period of nightwork (Knauth *et al.* 1978).

partners also report that their joint social life suffers as a result of shiftwork and that they experience 'high conflict' with their partner. Aspects of a spouse's homelife that alter while a partner is working shifts include being alone during the evening and nights, as well as having to keep noise-levels down after a night-shift has been worked. On some shift-schedules, workers may seldom see their young children for long periods of time, although when working morning- or night-shifts, they can pick up their children from school or support them in sports and after-school activities. Advantages of shift-work for the workers themselves, other than the usual financial gains, include increased use of banks and government offices during their stringent diurnal opening hours, as well as greater opportunities for some types of daytime recreation when most people are at work.

8.3.4 Shiftwork, sport, and recreation

Whether shiftwork is advantageous to participation in leisure pursuits seems to depend on the type of activity. In general, recreation based around the home (e.g. DIY, non-essential shopping) is facilitated whereas activities organized away from the home, including both watching and participating in sports, are hindered. Shiftworkers do not differ from the societal norm, in that they still would prefer to participate in leisure activities in the evenings and at the weekend (Hornberger and Knauth 1993). Such a desire may lead to some people leaving shiftwork; Herbert (1983) reported that individuals who had (or wished to) quit shiftwork stated that their leisure activities were disrupted to a greater degree than those who wished to remain working shifts. When past shiftworkers are asked to rate their reasons for needing to revert to daywork, 'better leisure-time possibilities' is rated as highly as 'could not adjust to the constant changes in shifts' and 'more time for the family' (Frese and Okonek 1984).

It is clear that some shiftworkers are involved in leisure-time physical activity. In fact, it is very unusual for some of one's recreational team-mates or clubmates not to be involved in some form of shiftwork. Atkinson (1994) found that 9 per cent of a sample of employed British competitive cyclists ($n = 97$) were shiftworkers, which is slightly lower than the minimum quoted for the general population.

A significant factor which has not been examined is the type of sports activity chosen. Although shiftwork interferes with conventional leisure pursuits requiring social contact, there may be increased opportunity to pursue individual sports, private hobbies, and domestic projects. To illustrate this, it was stated above that the proportion of competitive cyclists who were shiftworkers was slightly smaller than the rate reported for the general population. Cycling is one sport in which shiftworkers are not as disadvantaged as those involved in team sports; competitors can usually still train individually when they want to. In fact, it may be advantageous in some sports, for the shiftworker to be able to train in the hours of daylight which are not available to the dayworker in winter, as long as this does not interfere with any daytime sleep needed. This might mean that shiftworkers are over-represented in cycling compared to other sports, especially team sports. Individual sports, other than cycling, which may not be adversely affected by shiftwork, in terms of the opportunity for training times, are track and field athletics and swimming. Indeed, some British distance-runners have reached international standard while in shiftwork, though shiftwork may adversely affect their long-term running careers.

Although the opportunity for training may not be hindered by shiftwork in some sports, this training often cannot be scheduled in the early evening, which is the time of day thought to be optimum for training (Chapter 4). The opportunities for the shiftworker to participate in sports competitions are undoubtedly hindered, since these are most often scheduled in the early evening and at weekends. At these times, a shiftworker who has worked the previous night may be needing recuperative sleep. Even if the shiftworker does manage to arrive at the start of a competition, inappropriately phased rhythms, and/or marked sleep deprivation may adversely affect performance. Not surprisingly, if elite and professional athletes need to supplement their winnings with a conventional occupation, it seldom involves shiftwork. Ironically, those people who have been interested enough in sport and recreation to undertake degrees in sports studies or sports science and to gain employment in the leisure industry invariably find themselves working shifts, since the leisure demands of the general public peak outside normal working-hours. This may curtail their own leisure pursuits.

In summary, apart from home-based activities and the training for some individual sports, it appears that shiftworkers wish to perform leisure activities at the same times of day as dayworkers, but cannot. Participation in competitive sport, either as an individual or as part of team, is undoubtedly restricted by shiftwork, and for some people, this restriction becomes a significant factor in their cessation of shiftwork. Sport is one of the few leisure activities which may mediate long-term favourable changes in physiological functions and/or exacerbate the fatigue of the shiftworker. Physical activity performed at least twice a week is usually included in guidelines for improving shiftwork tolerance, but its usefulness is poorly understood and most shiftworkers do not seem to follow this advice (Wedderburn and Scholarios 1993). More research is needed, not only on how leisure interests are affected by shiftwork, but conversely on how leisure activities, especially those involving exercise affect tolerance to shiftwork (Section 8.6.3).

8.4 Shiftwork and health

Shiftwork is detrimental to some aspects of health, though the work-attendance record of shiftworkers is no worse than dayworkers. The role that prolonged circadian rhythm disturbance plays in any health deficits is unclear. For example, poorer health may result from a reduction in the amount of leisure-time physical activity while involved in shiftwork. It is clear, however, that 30–50 per cent of shiftworkers suffer from gastrointestinal disturbances, which is 2–5 times more than do dayworkers (Minors and Waterhouse 1981). This is probably linked to differences in the timing and composition of meals in shiftworkers. Although there is little evidence to suggest that shiftwork is associated with greater mortality rates, cardiovascular disorders appear to be more common in shiftworkers. There is also a growing concern that the fatigue and sleep disturbances experienced by shiftworkers may lead in some cases to chronic mental illhealth, such as depression.

A full discussion of shiftwork and health is beyond the scope of this book. Interested readers are directed to reviews by Minors and Waterhouse (1981) and Monk and Folkard (1992). Some effects on performance and its determinants are considered in the section that follows.

8.5 Shiftwork and performance

There is a tendency for accidents at work due to 'the human factor' to happen at night. For example, the human errors which resulted in the industrial accidents at Three-Mile-Island, Chernobyl, and Bopahl, occurred during the night-shift. However, such events should be interpreted with caution, as increased errors or accidents at night may result from poor lighting and because there is usually just a 'skeleton staff' present who may be less supervized than the dayworkers.

A differentiation can be made between sports performance and the ability to carry out industrial tasks, in that it is very unusual for the latter to include maximal exertion. In terms of physical performance, the ability to sustain submaximal exercise is most important for the shiftworker. However, other performance variables may be important for the shiftworker who wishes to compete in sport outside work. The mental performance components most relevant to shiftwork are simple perceptual–motor tasks and cognitive tasks, such as short-term memory. In addition, occupational tasks can be compromised by on-shift lapses in attention, which can of course be extremely dangerous.

8.5.1 Attention and mood states

Monk and Folkard (1992) cited three studies which show decreased attention during night-shifts. These were investigations into the frequency of 'nodding-off' while driving, the frequency of train drivers missing warning signals, and the frequency of minor accidents in hospital, which are all of course critically important. Again, differences between shifts in staffing levels and environmental conditions restrict the interpretation of results from these field studies. It cannot therfore be concluded that a worse performance at night is due completely to inappropriately phased circadian rhythms.

Mood variables may be important factors governing shiftwork performance, since negative mood states may lead to irresponsible behaviour or communication problems with work colleagues. Bohle and Tilley (1993) examined the effects of working night-shifts on six profile-of-mood states (POMS). 'Vigour' decreased and 'fatigue' increased on the fourth or fifth night-shifts compared to the baseline of daywork. These mood states are closely linked to the variables of arousal and sleepiness, respectively. Other, more antisocial mood states, such as anger, tension and depression, were unaffected by nightwork, suggesting that a shiftworker's tiredness on the night-shift does not seem to manifest itself in hostile thoughts. Conversely, there may be a great 'esprit de corps' within the small close-knit team that works the night-shift.

8.5.2 Mental performance

At least on the first few consecutive night-shifts, it is apparent that, perceptual–motor tasks, such as simple reaction-time, are worse than on a day-shift. This is in agreement with the circadian variation examined in subjects following a normal sleep–wake cycle (Monk and Folkard 1992). This performance in simple tasks adjusts slowly to successive nightwork, in parallel with the slow rate of change in the rhythm of body temperature (Fig. 8.1). Adjustment of the rhythm in hand-grip strength is also slow (Reinberg *et al.* 1980). While most shiftwork studies have examined simple tasks, real industrial tasks are increasingly of a more complex, cognitive nature. For example, workers are no longer ultimately responsible for the measurement and control of industrial processes 'by hand'. Instead, they operate and maintain electronic and pneumatic hardware and computer software, which together are more efficient than a human at the tasks. Performance rhythms in complex tasks with a high memory load (e.g. a six-target visual-search task) adjust faster to an eight-hour shift in the sleep–wake cycle than does the body-temperature rhythm (Folkard and Monk 1992).

Performance rhythms quickly readjust to a day-oriented routine on rest days between night-shift bouts, though even with more complex tasks, readjustment is not immediate. Reaction-time is impaired during the first day-off after a series of night-shifts, as are performances on a test of short-term memory (Meijman *et al*. 1993). Performances on the latter test were further impaired when subjects exercised to exhaustion on a cycle ergometer after the period of nightwork. Sleep deprivation over the period of nightwork would probably have some influence on performance during rest days.

8.5.3 Submaximal exercise performance

There is a wealth of literature concerning the effects of shiftwork on mental performance, but much less research has been done on how shiftwork affects the ability to perform physical work, either on-shift or during sports events in leisure-time. The physiological responses to shifwork have been measured by some authors (Bonnet 1990, for further reading and references). They speculated that glycogen and lipid stores are reduced on a night-shift, limiting the ability to perform long bouts of physical work at that time. It is extremely difficult to employ such physiological responses to exercise as indices of performance during shiftwork, since they are influenced by many factors including age, physical fitness, and time of day *per se*. This difficulty was illustrated by the results of Ostberg (1973) and Costa and Gaffuri (1975) who both measured the reliatioship between perceived exertion (RPE) and heart rate using cycle ergometry on different shifts. They found that, for a given level of RPE, heart rate was lower on the night-shift. Since lower heart-rate responses to exercise are found with aged subjects, Ostberg (1973) concluded that subjects are less fit and behave as if they are 'older' on the night-shift. There are problems with this interpretation. First, such rapid changes in the physiological responses to exercise should not be referred to as fluctuations in physical fitness, which usually denotes long-term, relatively stable, physiological adaptation. Second, a lower heart rate for a given level of exercise is usually associated with higher physical fitness. Thus, the results of these studies could be interpreted as indicating a *higher* exercise capability on the night-shift. This underlines the danger of using physiological responses to exercise to assess shiftwork performance. Submaximal responses may, however, still be useful for examining an individual's adjustment to shiftwork, since there is circadian rhythmicity in such responses. For example, Costa and Gaffuri (1975) found that minute ventilation, oxygen consumption, and expired carbon dioxide during exercise did not differ between morning-, afternoon- and evening-shifts when measured on the last sixth day of each series of shifts. It is not clear whether this indicates adjustment of the variables to the shiftwork, as the variables were not monitored every day of each shift that was worked.

More appropriate indices of work performance during shiftwork may be psychophysical tests, such as self-paced lifting of weights or self-chosen work-rate on a cycle ergometer (Chapter 4). Such indices of physical performance should be examined periodically over the entire duration of the workshift, since extrapolation of performance over short work-periods to longer durations is not reliable.

It is likely that the circadian performance rhythms of the shiftworker are not always fully entrained to a diurnal existence on days off, unlike dayworkers. This means that the shiftworking athlete may be attempting to perform optimally in sport with inappropriately phased rhythms. In a similar way to the athlete who has crossed time-zones, such performances are likely to be impaired, though for the shiftworker who is constantly changing shifts, circadian rhythms may never be fully entrained to a diurnal existence but may be constantly disturbed.

8.6 How can chronobiology help in alleviating the problems of shiftwork?

A knowledge of chronobiology can help people cope with shiftwork by consideration of the three main ergonomic interventions. These are:

(1) selection of shifworkers;
(2) task redesign (modification of shift schedules);
(3) the adoption of coping strategies by workers.

It is stressed that the chronobiological solution to a particular shift-work-related problem may compromise how another shiftwork stressor is dealt with. This is one reason why tolerance to shiftwork is examined from a multifactorial perspective, as shown by the "standard shiftwork index", a comprehensive measurement tool used in shiftwork research.

8.6.1 Selection of shiftworkers

There are several personal factors which are thought to be related to increased problems when attempting to work shifts. These include being aged over 50 years, being a morning-type person, being relatively inflexible with respect to sleep-times, and being physically unfit. It is stressed that persons with any of the above characteristics should not be immediately discounted from shift work. Each factor varies in its controllability and interacts with many other shift work factors. A good example of this is the effects of age on tolerance to shiftwork. Although older people find it easier to nap at times when body temperature is relatively high during the day, aged workers are less tolerant to shiftwork. From a chronobiological perspective, it is not so clear how age affects the adjustment of circadian rhythms during shiftwork. According to Aschoff's law (Aschoff 1981), the speed of entrainment of a circadian rhythm to a new sleep – close in wake schedule is inversely related to the amplitude of the rhythm. This suggests that the circadian rhythms of older subjects, with their smaller amplitudes, will allow an easier phase-adjustment process for the elderly. However, shiftwork becomes more, rather than less, difficult with age. Possible explanations for this may be that age-related disturbances in sleep far outweigh any benefits in faster entrainment rates when shiftwork is carried out, and rapid adjustments of circadian rhythms may be disadvantageous in modern, rapidly rotating, shift systems. Older subjects may also be less tolerant to nightwork because they are often found to be morning-type individuals with phase-advanced circadian rhythms. The phase-advance in the body-temperature rhythm of older individuals may increase the difficulty of day-sleep following night-duty. In agreement with this is the fact that high scores of 'morningness', independent of age, are associated with a poor tolerance to shiftwork in general. This may, however, depend greatly on the timing of the shift that is worked. It could be argued that, since the circadian rhythms of aged individuals are phase-advanced, older shiftworkers would be most effectively employed on earlier shifts (e.g. 06:00–14:00) than younger workers. More research is needed to confirm this hypothesis.

It is contentious whether women find it harder to cope with shiftwork than men. Their ability to cope seems to depend more on whether or not they succumb to the social pressures of fulfilling household and childcare roles, rather than on any chronobiological sex differences. Women do tend to sleep more than men, but when measures of actual shiftwork tolerance are recorded, invariably no differences between the sexes are noted. Oginska *et al.* (1993) found slightly better shiftwork tolerance in women over 50 years compared to younger females or males of a similar age. This may illustrate the influence of the degree of childcare responsibilities on shiftwork tolerance in younger women. Alternatively, there may be a positive effect associated with the cessation of the menstrual cycle (menopause), which occurs in middle-age.

The benefits of physical fitness for the dayworker are well-known. These include improved physical and mental health, which translates into less absenteeism from work and possibly better performance 'on the job'. Some studies have examined the effects of physical activity on the adjustment of circadian rhythms following changes in the sleep–wake cycle. These investigations are discussed in the section on coping startegies. Such isolated bouts of exercise during shiftwork should be examined separately from the adoption of prolonged physical training during shiftwork, which induces long-term physiological adaptation. Only a small amount of research has examined whether physical fitness *per se* (i.e. as an individual difference) affects circadian rhythms and tolerance to shiftwork and nightwork. In Chapter 4, it was stated that the rhythm amplitudes of physically fit subjects are 1.5 times higher than in unfit individuals, when they are studied under standardized laboratory conditions (Fig. 4.10). Fit individuals are more aroused and perform better during the day than unfit individuals, but show greater declines in these variables at night (i.e. rhythm amplitudes are greater). Thus, the differences in performance between fit and unfit people are reduced at night. The implications for shiftwork of these findings are unclear. Reinberg *et al.* (1980) found a positive correlation between the amplitude in body-temperature rhythm and tolerance to rapidly rotating shiftwork, but a negative correlation between rhythm amplitude and the entrainment rates to this type of shiftwork. However, the rhythm parameters were assessed while working shiftwork. This would have masked the nychthemeral rhythm characteristics. For example, it is possible that high-amplitude rhythms in tolerant shiftworkers are due to a greater regularity in the habits of sleep and wakefulness while working shiftwork.

8.6.2 Chronobiological design of shift systems

There are three main types of shift systems:

(1) rapidly-rotating shifts (2–3 days per shift);
(2) weekly rotating shifts (5–7 days per shift);
(3) permanent shifts (no rotation, but relatively stable times of one shift, interrupted only by rest days).

There is much debate concerning whether rapidly rotating shifts are better than permanent shifts. It is clear that weekly (slowly) rotating shift-schedules should be avoided, since a new workshift is adopted after significant, but not total, circadian adjustment has taken place. Thus, workers on weekly rotating shifts may find themselves in a perpetual 'state of flux', their rhythms never being fully entrained to a work–sleep schedule. Intuitively, rapidly rotating shifts are preferable since they do not allow significant circadian adjustment, they avoid the chronic sleep deprivation that is associated with long periods of consecutive night-shifts, and they are less disruptive to social and sports interests. However, they might be the worst system for optimizing occupational performance on shift (see below).

There are also people who choose to work permanent night-shifts and who do not experience any significant difficulties. Reasons for this may be higher wages, a preference for minimal supervision which is a characteristic of the night-shift, and a liking for the favourable working 'atmosphere' sometimes found in a close-knit night-shift team. Permanent nightwork may be the best schedule for extreme evening-types, though it is not known whether such people gravitate towards permanent nightwork or adapt to it extremely well. Whatever the permanent nightworkers' attributes are, they are unlikely to be keen on competitive sport since their participation would be severely limited.

It was stated earlier that many performance rhythms are slow to adjust to a change in the sleep – wake cycle. From a performance and safety perspective, permanent nightwork may therefore be superior to rapidly rotating schedules, as the former is associated with the greatest adjustment of performance rhythms. It may be that the cumulative sleep loss associated with permanent nightwork would offset any benefits from well-adjusted circadian rhythms. Figure 8.1 shows that circadian rhythms do not fully entrain to even a large number of consecutive night-shifts. This would be exacerbated if workers readily returned to a diurnal existence on their days off. Consequently, Folkard (1992) maintained that for optimum safety and efficiency in critical industries and services, a small amount of permanent nightwork is necessary, but ideally, a nocturnal subsociety would have to exist in which workers remain nocturnally active on their days off. To summarize, slowly rotating shifts have disadvantages. The debate about rapid versus permanent rotation will continue until there are more well-controlled studies that directly compare the two shift systems.

The direction of work-shift rotation has also been analysed chronobiologically. Since the endogenous clock shows a period of greater than 24 h, the human circadian system adjusts more slowly to phase-advances than to phase-delays in the work – sleep schedule. Thus, for the traveller (Chapters 6 and 7), subjective symptoms are less on travelling westwards compared to eastwards. For the shiftworker, this means that shifts are better rotated in a forward direction (morning – afternoon – night) than backwards. It is unclear whether there is an interaction between the direction and speed of rotation.

The timing of shifts within a shift system may vary considerably from the conventional 06:00–14:00, 14:00–22.00, and 22:00–06:00. The starting time of the morning-shift may be critical (and also affects the starting times of the other shifts, assuming the work-periods are the same). The start of the morning-shift should be as late as possible since this encourages longer sleep-times (workers do not seem to retire to bed unusually early before a morning-shift). There is also less fatigue (and a reduced likelihood of accidents) on a late-starting morning-shift. It is stressed that a compromise must be reached between the lateness of the morning-shift and the lateness of sleep following the night-shift, since it is more difficult to sleep when body temperature is rising in the morning. This compromise may take the form of longer morning- or afternoon-shifts and a shortened night-shift.

8.6.3 Chronobiological coping strategies

Guidelines on coping strategies for shiftworkers are the least researched, but potentially the most fruitful element of ergonomic intervention. Although many studies have described the problems associated with shiftwork and identified individual differences in tolerance to shiftwork, few researchers have considered how individuals cope with shiftwork. This is so, even though shiftworkers do not necessarily adopt through experience what are considered the best coping strategies as a result of scientific findings (Wedderburn and Scholarios 1993).

Chronobiological coping strategies are centred around obtaining the correct zeitgeber information (Chapter 1) at appropriate times of the solar day. This will depend mostly on the type of shift system. During permanent or slowly rotating shifts, zeitgebers should be directed towards ensuring circadian rhythms peak during worktime (at night), even on full days off. During rapidly rotating shifts, minimal circadian adjustment to nightwork is required so that a diurnal existence can be maintained. Ideally any chronobiological coping strategy, should not impinge detrimentally on other aspects of the shift worker's life (e.g. social and domestic situations). A fuller discussion is provided by Monk and Folkard (1992). Nevertheless, the main potential zeitgebers in humans are sleep, activity, bright light, meals, and social factors.

A worker on a rapidly rotating system should be exposed to bright light as much as possible during the day (except during sleep) and should avoid a heavy meal during the night-shift. A short sleep taken on the longest break of the night-shift might also help to 'anchor' sleep to the nocturnal hours. The benefits of this should of course be weighed up against a possible decrease in alertness during the night-shift. Coping strategies are harder to implement for the permanent night-worker, the major difficulty being optimizing the timing of zeitgebers on days off. Night-workers should try to sleep as soon as possible after the night-shift and should avoid naps in the evening or in work breaks (i.e. they should try to avoid 'anchor' sleeps). Ideally, the night-worker should be exposed to bright light during occupational work and should be in a completely dark environment during sleep. The realization of this impinges on both the employer and the home. Family life would also be affected by the recommendation that permanent nightworkers should try to remain nocturnal on their days off. A compromise may be that workers should remain in bed as long as possible in the morning and retire to bed as late as they can.

The use of physical exercise as a strategy for coping with shiftwork is extremely complicated due to the fact that it can mediate: (1) favourable training responses that increase physical working capacity; (2) fatigue and; (3) masking effects on circadian rhythms.

There is also increasing evidence that physical activity acts as a zeitgeber in humans and animals, influencing the endogenous component of circadian rhythms.

Harma *et al.* (1988) examined the effects of physical training intervention on female shiftworkers. During the training period, there was a reduction in general fatigue and musculoskeletal symptoms during shiftwork and in fatigue while working the nightshift, although fatigue increased on the evening-shift (the shift worked after the training session) (Fig. 8.2).

Although maximal oxygen consumption ($\dot{V}O_2$ max) was increased after 4 months of training, there was a decrease in the amplitude of the body-temperature rhythm (Figure 8.2).

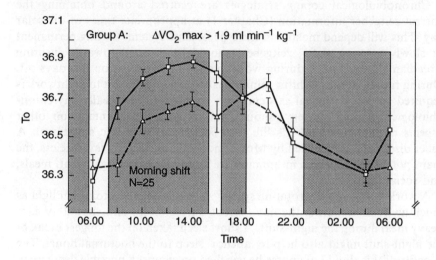

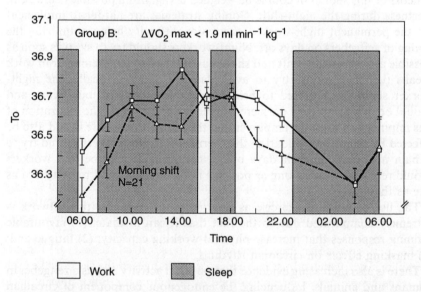

Fig. 8.2 Effects of physical training on the circadian rhythm of oral temperature while working a morning-shift. Group A showed an increase in $\dot{V}O_2$max following physical training of more than 1.9 ml min^{-1} kg.$^{-1}$. Group B showed an increase in $\dot{V}O_2$max of less than this value. The full line is before training and the dashed line after training (Harma *et al.* 1988).

There is some evidence that physical activity acts as a zeitgeber. For example, during constant wakefulness over 24 hours the acrophase of the body-temperature rhythm occurs slightly earlier in the solar day after a programme of morning exercise, but later than usual after several days of evening exercise (Piercy and Lack 1988). Thus an earlier phasing of body temperature should be useful for optimizing performance during a morning-shift but will be disadvantageous during shifts in the afternoon or at night. Behavioural factors (including exercise) have been found to influence the phases of circadian rhythms in animal research. Although such zeitgeber actions of exercise have yet to be confirmed in humans, the effects of 90 minutes of exercise on entrainment rates of body temperature following a shift in the sleep-wake cycle of a worker have been studied (Schmidt *et al.* 1990). Circadian phase was recorded on the second bout of nightwork and compared to that recorded in normal daywork. The activity period was carried out on the first duty of nightwork. The results indicated that activity accelerated the rate of entrainment to nightwork. Whether any masking effects of the exercise were 'carried over' to the second night-shift needs to be known before any definite conclusions can be drawn.

8.6 Overview

The number of people participating in shiftwork is substantial. Despite methodological constraints on experiments in the workplace, shiftwork research has identified three sources of strain which may be related to the slightly poorer health of shiftworkers. First, many circadian rhythms adjust slowly following changes in the sleep-wake cycle. Some never fully adjust to nightwork. Second, shiftworkers get less sleep which is of a poorer quality than dayworkers. Third, shiftwork can interfere significantly with family and social life. Shiftworkers wish to, but cannot, perform leisure activities at the same times of day as dayworkers. For people with solitary hobbies or those training for (but not competing in) individual sports, this may not be a problem. For those participating in team sports or any type of competitive sport, this restriction may become one of the major factors in their leaving shiftwork.

The performance rhythms most relevant to industrial contexts are those of complex tasks, which adjust more rapidly to changes in the sleep–wake cycle than the simple tasks of reaction-time or grip strength. Since physiological responses to exercise cannot be used reliably as performance indices during shiftwork, more research is needed to identify how submaximal work is paced throughout different shifts. Although, morning-type individuals may find nightwork more difficult than evening-types, they could be suited to early morning-shifts. Physical fitness or activity improves certain aspects of shiftwork tolerance, but more research is needed to identify the optimum amount, frequency, and timing of leisure-time exercise during shiftwork. Differences in gender or circadian rhythm characteristics should not be used on their own to select shiftworkers. All shift-schedules should be rotated in the forward direction. Slowly rotating (e.g. weekly) shift-schedules should be avoided. Although rapidly rotating systems are the most popular schedules, a minority of people may prefer permanent nightwork. Coping strategies for shiftworkers are centred around obtaining the correct zeitgeber information (e.g. light, meals, sleep, activity) at the appropriate times of day.

Further reading

Bonnet M. H. (1990). Dealing with shift-work: physical fitness, temperature and napping. *Work and Stress* **4**, 261–74.

Harma, M. I., Ilmarinen, J., Knauth, P., Rutenfranz, J., and Hanninen, P. (1988). Physical training intervention in shift-workers. 1. The effects of intervention on fitness, fatigue, sleep, and psychomotor symptoms. *Ergonomics*, **31**, 39–50.

Monk, T. H. and Folkard, S. (1992). *Making shift-work tolerable*. Taylor and Francis, Basingstoke.

Minors, D. S. and Waterhouse, J. (1981). *Circadian rhythms and the human*. Wright, London.

References

Aschoff, J. (ed.). (1981). *Biological rhythms. Handbook of behavioural neurobiology*. Plenum Press, New York.

Atkinson, G. (1994). *Effects of age on human circadian rhythms in physiological and performance measures*. (Unpublished doctoral thesis.) Liverpool John Moores University.

Baumgart, P., Walger, P., Fuchs, G., Dorst, K. G., Vetter, H., and Rahn, K. H. (1989). Twenty-four-hour blood pressure is not dependent on endogenous circadian rhythm. *J. Hyperten.*, **7**, 331–4.

Bohle, P., and Tilley, A. J. (1993). Predicting mood change on night shift. *Ergonomics*, **36**, 125–34.

Costa, G. and Gaffuri, E. (1975). Studies of perceived exertion rate on bicycle ergometer in conditions reproducing some aspects of industrial work (shift-work, noise). In *Physical work and effort* (ed. G. Borg), pp. 297–306. Pergamon Press, Oxford.

Folkard, S. (1992). Is there a 'best compromise' shift system? *Ergonomics*, **35**, 1453–63.

Frese, M. and Okenek, K. (1984). Reasons to leave shift-work and psychological and psychosomatic complaints of former shift-workers. *J. Appl. Physiol.*, **69**, 509–14.

Harma, M. I., Ilmarinen, J., Knauth, P., Rutenfranz, J., and Hanninen, P. (1988). Physical training intervention in shift-workers. 1. The effects of intervention on fitness, fatigue, sleep, and psychomotor symptoms. *Ergonomics*, **31**, 39–50.

Herbert, A. (1983). The influence of shift-work on leisure activities. A study with repeated measurement. *Ergonomics*, **26**, 565–74.

Hornberger, S. and Knauth, P. (1993). Interindividual differences in the subjective valuation of leisure time utility. *Ergonomics*, **36**, 255–64.

Knauth, P., Rutenfranz, J., Herrmann, G., and Poppel, S. (1978). Re-entrainment of body temperature in experimental shift-work studies. *Ergonomics*, **21**, 775–83.

Meijman, T., van der Meer, O., and van Dormolen, M. (1993). The after-effects of night-work on short-term memory performance. *Ergonomics*, **36**, 37–42.

Minors, D. S. and Waterhouse, J. (1981). *Circadian rhythms and the human*. Wright, London.

Monk, T. H. and Folkard, S. (1992). *Making shift-work tolerable*, pp. 1–2. Taylor and Francis, Basingstoke.

Oginska, H., Pokorski, J., and Oginska, A. (1993). *Gender, ageing and shift-work intolerance*. *Ergonomics*, **36**, 161–8.

Ostberg, O. (1973). Interindividual differences in circadian fatigue patterns of shift-workers. *Brit. J. Indust. Med.*, **30**, 341–51.

Piercy, J., and Lack, L. (1988). Daily exercise can shift the endogenous circadian rhythm. *Sleep Res.*, **17**, 393.

Reinberg, A., Andlauer, P., Guillet, P., and Nicolai, A. (1980). Oral temperature, circadian rhythm amplitude, ageing and tolerance to shift-work. *Ergonomics*, **23**, 55–64.

Roberts, K. and Chambers, D. A. (1985). Changing 'times'. Hours of work/patterns of leisure. *World Leis. Recreat. Assoc.*, **27**, 17–23.

Scherrer, J. (1981). Man's work and circadian rhythm through the ages. In *Night and shift-work: biological and social aspects* (ed. A. Reinberg, N. Vieux, and P. Andlauer), pp. 1–10. Pergamon Press, Oxford.

Schmidt, K. P., Koehler, W. K., Fleissner, G., and Pfug, B. (1990). Locomotor activity accelerates the adjustment of the temperature rhythm in shift-work. *J. Interdiscipl. Cycle Res.*, **21**, 243–5.

Smith, L. and Folkard, S. (1993). The perceptions and feelings of shift-workers' partners. *Ergonomics*, **36**, 299–306.

Wedderburn, A. and Scholarios, D. (1993). Guidelines for shift-workers: trials and errors? *Ergonomics*, **36**, 211–18.

Young, B. M. (1982). The shift towards shiftwork. *New Society*, **61**, 96–7.

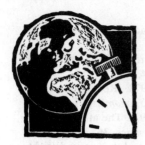

9
The menstrual cycle and exercise

9.1 Introduction

In ancient civilizations, it was thought that extraordinary natural phenomena accompanied historic human events, such as births, deaths, and battles and it was also usual to link such occurrences with the phases of the moon. The effects of the lunar tide are more evident in marine than in human life. Nevertheless, rhythms with a period of about a month exist and are known as circamensal. The most obvious human rhythm of this length is the female menstrual cycle, although there is no link between the lunar cycle and the menstrual cycle.

Female reproduction processes include the production of ova and cyclical changes in both ovaries and uterus. A single egg is released each month by the ovaries which enters the uterine or fallopian tube. If fertilized by sperm from a male partner, it is nurtured by nutrients from uterine cytoplasm until it is implanted within the womb where it develops. Unfertilized eggs degenerate. This biological cycle, evident from puberty until the menopause when it disappears, underpins the reproduction of the human species.

In this chapter, the physiological factors regulating the menstrual cycle are described and the potential effects of the physiological changes on performance of physical activity are considered. The normal menstrual cycle may be disturbed due to various factors, such as diet, stress, and strenuous exercise. Some individuals suffer discomfort more than others at particular phases of the menstrual cycle, for which they require treatment. Strenuous exercise can eliminate the menstrual cycle and may cause large decreases in circulating reproductive hormones. These changes interact with the woman's health, as well as with her exercise capability, and these interactions are discussed towards the end of the chapter. Some attention is given also to the physiological changes that occur when the cycle ceases during pregnancy and for some months after term.

9.2 The normal menstrual cycle

The normal menstrual cycle has an average cycle length of 28 days, but varies between individuals and between cycles from 23–38 days. Menses (menstruation) lasts 4–5 days during which about 40 ml of blood is discharged with about two-thirds of the endometrial lining. Menstruation refers to shedding of the surface portion of the endometrial wall and the bleeding that accompanies it. Blood losses usually vary from 25–65 ml, but can exceed 200 ml, when the individual may be anaemic as a result of the heavy loss of blood. The endometrial wall is renewed under the influence of oestrogens (mainly oestradiol), while follicle-stimulating hormone (FSH) promotes the maturation of an ovum into a graafian follicle. This ovulates at about midcycle (day 14), with ovulation being triggered by a surge of luteinizing hormone (LH). The ovum has to be fertilized within 24 hours for conception to occur. The wall of the ruptured follicle, from which the ovum has burst, then collapses, and the follicle now forms the corpus luteum which produces increased amounts of progesterone, and which characterizes the luteal phase. The corpus luteum regresses if implantation has not occurred, usually by day 21, and progesterone levels fall premenses. Thus, the main function of progesterone is to prepare the uterine lining for implantation of the fertilized ovum. The endometrium regresses and is shed in menses with the start of the next cycle.

The menstrual cycle is regulated by a complex system incorporating the hypothalamus (gonadotrophin-releasing factor or GnRH), anterior pituitary (FSH and LH), the ovaries, follicles, and corpus luteum (oestrogens, progesterone and inhibin) with feedback loops to the pituitary and to the hypothalamus. Contraceptive pills, composed of oestrogen and progesterone combinations, prevent ovulation by inhibiting LH release. The whole control system is referred to as the hypothalamic–pituitary–ovarian axis (Fig. 9.1).

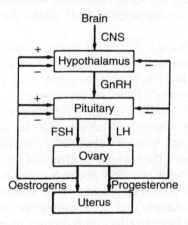

Fig. 9.1 The hypothalamic–pituitary–ovarian axis.

The several hormones coordinate the functions of the uterus with those of the ovaries very closely within the overall menstrual cycle. At the end of menses, the endometrium undergoes a proliferative phase under the influence of oestradiol and progesterone. Oestradiol stimulates development of the surface portion of the endometrium and the spiral arteries. At ovulation, progesterone causes the endometrium to develop mucous glands and secrete mucus, and endometrial cells to accumulate glycogen in preparation for a fertilized ovum. As the ovum reaches the uterus, the follicular cells form the corpus luteum which secretes large quantities of oestrogen (oestradiol) and progesterone. These hormones act by negative feedback to suppress the release of GnRH, FSH, and LH. If the fertilized ovum is implanted in the uterus, progesterone maintains the endometrium and inhibits uterine contractions during pregnancy.

As mentioned earlier, events in ovarian phases are tied in with the thickening and shedding of the endometrium. The period of bleeding is followed by the follicular phase of the ovarian cycle. Both FSH and LH remain nearly constant until a peak in oestradiol secretion occurs on the day before ovulation. Oestradiol acts by positive feedback to cause a rise in LH and GnRH which then stimulates both LH and FSH. The result is a pronounced surge in LH and a lesser elevation in FSH.

After ovulation in midcycle, the ovarian events are characterized by the luteal phase. Progesterone levels further increase, causing the secretory phase of the endometrial cycle. If implantation does not occur, the corpus luteum regresses, oestrogen and progesterone drop to their lowest levels, and GnRH, FSH, and LH are freed from negative feedback. The sloughing of the endometrial lining is initiated by the large fall in progesterone which causes blood-vessel spasms, ischaemia, and necrosis of the surface endometrial cells. This late luteal phase is known as premenses. As menstruation begins, follicle development under the influence of FSH marks the start of the next cycle (Fig. 9.2).

Many hormonal changes during the course of the normal menstrual cycle influence other aspects of human physiology that are important in exercise performance. There is a rise in core temperature of about 0.5 °C coinciding with ovulation. Bodyweight increases premenses due to the storage of water and altered potassium: sodium ratios. Weight loss starts with menses. Some women suffer severe abdominal cramps due to increased prostaglandin production premenses. Administration of prostaglandin inhibitors helps to reduce this problem – the lowered incidence of menstrual-related stomach cramp noted in athletes is probably due to lowered levels of prostaglandins. Others suffer painful menstruation known as dysmenorrhoea. In addition, the many hormonal changes that occur during the menstrual cycle can alter metabolism and thus have an effect on responses to exercise. Furthermore it is possible that the elevations in steroid hormones (oestrogen and progesterone) affect muscular strength in an analogous manner to the steroids used illegally by some athletes.

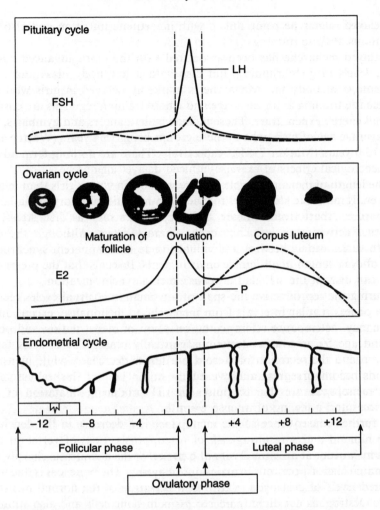

Fig. 9.2 The ovarian and endometrical phases during the menstrual cycle.

9.3 Menarche and the menopause

The appearance of menstrual flow for the first time signals the culmination of development of the female reproductive system. This is known as menarche and is a major biological marker of growth and development. It occurs on average at about 12.8 years in girls in the USA and 13.0 years in the UK, though there is wide individual variation. There is a gradual increase in GnRH from about the eighth year of life, but the onset of puberty (menarche) is probably triggered by maturation processes occurring else-where in the brain rather than by the hypothalamus. There is some evidence of delayed menarche being linked with inadequate nutrition and also with strenuous athletic training.

Delayed menarche has been associated with the more advanced competitive levels in girls' running, but also with a low body mass and a low percentage of body fat. Menarche is markedly delayed in girls who start systematic training at an early age and whose training regimens are costly in overall energy expenditure. These include ballet dancers and gymnasts, with the average age of menarche in these groups being 15.4 years (Warren 1980) and 15.0 years (Marker 1981), respectively. There are no long-term adverse gynaecological effects of exercise-induced delayed menarche.

The length of menstrual cycle is more variable in young girls than in adult women. It may take some years for the hypothalamic–pituitary–gonadal axis to mature. Apart from athletes' training, factors such as diet, stress, and habitual activity can influence cyclic characteristics. Although the cycle length varies widely between individuals, there is an apparent synchronization of cycle length in all-female environments. It seems that the presence of men can disrupt the signals that cause such a synchronization.

During the reproductive life-span of a woman, menstrual cycles recur at more or less regular intervals from menarche to menopause, except during pregnancy. Menopause refers to the cessation of menstruation and occurs around age 50 as ovarian functions gradually cease. The follicles fail to develop and the secretion of steroid hormones decreases, while menstrual periods become irregular and eventually stop. The 'hot flushes' associated with menopause are due to pulses in LH producing dilatation of skin arterioles and a feeling of intense warmth.

A further consequence of the menopause is a decrease in the density or bone mineral and a resulting risk of osteoporosis. Loss of vertebral bone mass may occur at an annual rate of 6 per cent which contrasts sharply with an annual loss of 1 per cent in males due to ageing. The bone loss is due to the lowered levels of oestrogens that follow cessation of the normal menstrual cycle. Oestrogens act directly on receptors in bone cells and also stimulate secretion of calcitonin from the thyroid gland. This hormone maintains the integrity of bone by lowering blood calcium and moving it to bone. It also blocks the actions of parathyroid hormone: both hormones regulate bone homeostasis by balancing bone formation and bone reabsorption. In the growing skeleton, more bone is formed than is reabsorbed, but the remodelling of bone is in equilibrium in the adult. The regular remodelling of bone occurs over a three-week period and, being similar in males and females, is independent of the menstrual cycle. After about 40 years of age, more bone is reabsorbed than is formed, but this is accentuated in the female once oestrogen levels fall. Exercise and dietary calcium can attenuate bone losses. The most effective treatment is hormone-replacement therapy with oestrogens which has an additional benefit of protecting against coronary heart disease. A current controversy is that an increased risk of breast and endometrial cancer is thought to be associated with this treatment but incorporation of progestins is believed to reduce this risk.

Associated with the menopause, there is a range of symptoms, which may impinge on health and well-being. A change in insulin sensitivity increases the risk of diabetes, and an alteration in lipoprotein metabolism increases the risk of cardiovascular disease. The latter can be offset by oestrogen treatment. Hot flushes are acompanied by burning sensations and pressure in the head, increases in blood flow, and skin temperature. The fall in oestrogen levels leads to a decrease in beta-endorphins: as these substances are involved in thermoregulation, the control of body temperature may therefore be unstable, leading to 'hot flushes'.

9.4 Exercise during the menstrual cycle

In many cultures, there have been taboos attributed to the menstrual cycle, particularly menses. In the context of sport, menstruating women were discouraged from swimming for hygienic reasons, and for a long time it was thought that they should not take part at all in strenuous exercise. Indeed, the Olympic track and field programme was extended to 800 m only at the 1964 games in Tokyo. The first Olympic marathon race for women took place at the Los Angeles Games in 1984 and the first 10-km gold medal was contested by female runners at Seoul in 1988. Nowadays, female participation in sport is socially acceptable in most countries and menses is no bar to training or competing.

Retrospective studies of athletic performances have shown that Olympic gold medals have been won, and world records set, at all stages of the menstrual cycle. This indicates that exercise performance is not necessarily impaired during the menstrual cycle. Responses to submaximal exercise may be subject to changes, e.g. a rise in ventilation at a set exercise intensity has been reported during the luteal phase (O'Reilly and Reilly 1990). This rise was associated with the surge in progesterone noted at the same time and was also linked with a higher rating of exertion. This elevation in ventilation would increase CO_2 output, but does not seem to affect the maximal oxygen consumption ($\dot{V}O_2$ max), as determined by an incremental exercise-test to exhaustion.

The fuel utilised for oxidative metabolism can have a significant influence on performance in prolonged sustained exercise. In endurance athletic events lasting 90 min or more, the level of performance may be determined by prestart stores of glycogen in liver and muscle. Mechanisms that increase these depots or spare existing stores by increasing fat oxidation can enhance overall performance. The elevated levels of progesterone and oestrogen during the luteal phase of the menstrual cycle might benefit submaximal exercise of long duration by diminishing the utilization of glycogen. This view is corroborated by the finding of increased free fatty acids during exercise in the luteal phase (De Mendoza *et al.* 1979) and lowered levels of blood lactate (Jurowski-Hall *et al.* 1981). Amenorrheic athletes have a lower respiratory exchange ratio (RER) in mid-luteal compared to mid-follicular phases of the menstrual cycle during exercise at 35 per cent and 60 per cent of VO_2 max (Hackney *et al.* 1994). The mechanism for altering fuel utilisation is likely to be a hormone-sensitive lipase which promotes lipolysis and is activated by the hormonal changes in the luteal phase. The time-span over which performance might be enhanced is likely to be only a matter of 3–4 days, before progesterone falls premenses. This possible enhancement may be counteracted in a competitive context at other phases of the menstrual cycle when catecholamine secretion, which leads to similar effects, is increased in the course of competitive stress.

Potentially, low oestrogen levels have an adverse effect on human strength. The effect has been demonstrated in ovariectomized mice whose force production was impaired after surgery. The ergogenic effect of oestrogen has also been demonstrated in post-menopausal women when the adductor pollicies muscle (which draws the thumb in over the palm of the hand) was isolated for measurement of isometric force under experimental conditions (Phillips *et al.* 1993). The active stretch force – the tension within the muscle in response to its being stretched – is not impaired and the weakness can be offset by hormone-replacement therapy. This loss of strength in the muscles of ageing females may accentuate the loss in bone strength due to demineralization. A cyclical variation of muscle strength with changes in oestrogen levels during the normal menstrual cycle is difficult to show. This is because performance in gross muscular function is influenced by a variety of factors other than circulating hormones.

The quality of sports performance depends on psychological factors, such as attitude, motivation, and willingness to work hard. The dramatic effects of the menstrual cycle are observed in mood factors: positive moods are evident during the follicular and ovulatory phases, with negative moods being prominent preceding and during menses (Table 9.1). These variations should be recognized by sports coaches, who should take them into account in structuring the training programmes of female athletes.

Table 9.1 Profile of mood states at the four phases of the menstrual cycle (mean ± SD). A higher score means a greater tendency towards each mood description (O'Reilly and Reilly 1990).

	Menses	Follicular	Ovulatory	Luteal
Tension–anxiety	13.2 ± 3.4	8.2 ± 1.9	6.9 ± 2.5	14.4 ± 3.5
Depression	16.1 ± 6.7	8.1 ± 4.2	8.3 ± 5.1	17.4 ± 6.2
Anger–hostility	3.9 ± 10.0	4.4 ± 2.3	4.7 ± 3.4	7.4 ± 3.0
Vigour–activity	9.0 ± 2.4	16.2 ± 1.9	22.7 ± 1.3	12.2 ± 2.3
Fatigue–inertia	11.2 ± 2.8	5.5 ± 0.7	1.5 ± 0.7	10.4 ± 1.8
Confusion	9.1 ± 1.4	4.8 ± 1.0	2.8 ± 1.4	8.2 ± 2.0

Variations in mood are most pronounced in those who suffer from premenstrual tension (PMT). In its extreme form, it is characterized by irritability, aggression, abnormal behaviour, and confusion. Bouts of irritation may be affected by the time of day, linked with fluctuations in blood glucose, with irritability peaking in the late morning if breakfast is missed (Dalton 1978). In less extreme forms, sufferers may feel anxious and tired, but unable to relax. Although the incidence of PMT is probably less common in athletes than in nonparticipants in sport, women in general seem to be more susceptible than normal to injury during premenstrual days. A study of Swedish female soccer players showed that injury was most likely to occur immediately prior to menses (Möller-Nielsen and Hammar 1989).

9.5 Athletic amenorrhea

Female athletes on strenuous athletic training programmes are known to experience disruption of the normal menstrual cycle. One irregularity is a shortened luteal phase (Bonen *et al.* 1981). Secondary amenorrhea or absence of menses for a prolonged period, is also reported. So-called 'athletic amenorrhea' is linked with low levels of body fat, low body weight, and high training loads, while stress is also implicated.

Amenorrhea is associated with low values of body fat, though the responsible mechanism has not been clearly established. It is known that endurance training lowers body fat, which in turn leads to a reduced peripheral production of oestrogens through aromatization of androgens, catalysed by aromatase in fat cells. The peripheral production of oestrogens is thought to be important in stimulating the hypothalamic–pituitary–ovarian axis. Hard exercise or intentional weight reduction will lower pituitary FSH secretion, prevent follicular development and ovarian oestrogen secretion, and decrease progesterone secretion.

Exercise-induced amenorrhea occurs in 20 per cent of female athletes, compared to a prevalence of 5 per cent in the general population. In runners, the prevalence increases linearly with training mileage to nearly 50 per cent in all athletes covering 130 km (80 miles) per week. This linear increase is not found in swimmers and cyclists (Drinkwater 1986), as these athletes do not have to support their bodyweight during exercise and their bones are not subject to the same repetitive loads as in the runners.

A study of British athletes indicated that stress may also be implicated in the occurrence of amenorrhea (Reilly and Rothwell 1988). In this study, a sample of international, club, and recreational distance-runners was divided into those with amenorrheic, oligomenorrheic (irregular) or regular (normal) menstrual cycles. The amenorrheic athletes were younger and lighter, had less body fat, experienced more life stress, had a higher training mileage, and trained at a faster pace than the other groups (Table 9.2). A high frequency of competition was the most powerful discriminator of the amenorrheic individuals from the other groups. This finding supports the possibility that increased outputs of catecholamine, cortisol, and endorphins interfere with the normal menstrual cycle by affecting the hypothalamic–pituitary– ovarian axis. Training-induced amenorrhea does not necessarily mean the athlete is infertile. Ovulation can occur spontaneously and fertility can be restored after a long absence of menses. Exercise-related menstrual distur- bances are quickly reversed with a reduction of high training loads, and a marginal increase in body fat.

Table 9.2   Factors related to amenorrhea in a sample of British athletes (mean ± SD). (Reilly and Rothwell 1988.)

	Amenorrheic	Oligomenorrheic	Normal
Age (years)	25.4 (5.7)a	31.8 (7.3)	32.7 (6.6)
Body mass (kg)	50.0 (5.4)a	55.3 (3.9)	57.0 (6.9)
Body fat (%)	16.1 (4.3)b	27.5 (2.8)	25.6 (2.9)
Life stress/year	693 (393)a	286 (234)	494 (282)
Years running	6.0 (4.6)	5.0 (6.4)	5.3 (4.8)
Miles/week	55 (25)	44 (27)	34 (20)
Pace/mile (min)	7.0 (1.0)	7.6 (1.4)	7.9 (1.1)
Races/year	29.1 (14.0)a	9.1 (7.2)	16.3 (14.0)

a indicates $P < 0.05$, b $P < 0.01$ compared with normal.

9.6 Other problems associated with severe athletic training

It is known that trimming body-fat depots can enhance running performance because it decreases the load to be lifted repetitively against gravity. The extra fat of females is of no metabolic advantage, since the fat cannot be mobilized immediately for use by active muscles. Undue concern with losing bodyweight in highly trained runners can itself cause problems in the promotion of eating disorders such as anorexia.

There is an ultradian rhythm to the timing of our meals. The normal pattern of feeding fits in generally well with rhythms in gut motility. These rhythms are reinforced by a lack of appetite at nighttime when the body would normally be resting. Women overly concerned about their body image may develop abnormal eating behaviour that fluctuates between bingeing and starving. The most commonly reported eating disorders in athletes are anorexia and bulimia. The athletic groups most at risk are distance runners and gymnasts, though ballet dancers and aerobic enthusiasts are also affected. The result is a hormone imbalance with the consequent risk of malnutrition and bone demineralization.

Another contemporary concern is the effect of prolonged hypoestrogenic levels on bone mineralization. The loss of calcium from bone is associated with high training mileage and amenorrhea leading to vulnerability to stress fractures in the lower limbs. The lumbar vertebrae also exhibit decreased bone density and it seems that trabecular rather than cortical bone is mostly affected (Drinkwater 1988). The lowered spinal bone mass noted in young distance-runners resembles that observed in postmenopausal women and seems to be linked with the low oestrogen levels. Light athletes appear to be more vulnerable than heavier runners. Although a moderate level of exercise stimulates bone growth and reverses bone loss in older women, overtraining in younger runners leads to decreased bone density and stress fractures. Reducing the training load and decreasing the frequency of competitive racing helps to restore the normal menstrual cycle. However, the interactions between training parameters and a liability to osteoporosis have yet to be fully explored.

9.7 Oral contraceptive use

The reproductive process can be prevented by the oral administration of pills, known as oral contraceptives. These work by blocking the normal hormonal feedback mechanisms and inhibiting ovulation. Oral contraception may also be used to treat menstrual discomfort and to stabilize the menstrual cycle. Athletes may use oral contraceptives to ensure that important competitions do not coincide with menses.

The administration of oestrogen or progesterone in appropriate amounts in the follicular phase can prevent the preovulatory surge of LH secretion that triggers ovulation. Contraceptive pills contain combinations of oestrogen in small amounts and progestins (substances that mimic the actions of progesterone), since excess of either type of hormone can cause excessive bleeding. Medication is started early in the cycle and is continued beyond the time that ovulation would normally have taken place.

Administration can then be stopped to allow menstrual flow to occur as usual and a new cycle to commence. The use of contraceptive pills demonstrates that the menstrual cycle is produced by a series of feedback loops rather than originating from some internal master bodyclock (see Chapter 1).

There is disagreement about whether or not oral contraception affects the performance of exercise. The adverse effects of body-water retention may have been due to the particular combination of hormones used in early contraceptive pills. However, if use of the contraceptive pill prevents adverse menstrual effects, the result is going to be beneficial. Their main influence is probably that performance is more consistent than normal, since they stabilize the fluctuations in peptide and steroid hormone concentrations linked with the menstrual cycle.

9.8 Exercise during pregnancy

Pronounced physiological changes during pregnancy impinge on exercise performance or the continuance of training. These include altered hormonal concentrations, particularly progesterone and human chorionic gonadotrophin (hCG), increased plasma volume, and red blood cells, increased ventilatory response, and associated changes in pCO_2, the partial pressure of carbon dioxide in the blood. Bodyweight increases during pregnancy, so altering the woman's centre of gravity. The average weight gain during pregnancy is about 10 kg, with the gain being slowest in the first trimester.

Pregnancy itself does not prohibit the performance of exercise. There have been cases of top athletes competing in the London Marathon while pregnant, and medals were won at the 1956 Olympics in Melbourne by pregnant athletes. Indeed, it is likely that women runners would race in the first trimester before the pregnancy is detected. The American athlete, Karen Cosgrove, completed a marathon in 2 h 46 min. in her first month of pregnancy. She maintained a distance of 100–130 km (60–80 miles) per week until 36 weeks. She did 60 min exercise on a cycle ergometer on the day before giving birth to a healthy 3.35 kg boy (Higdon 1981).

Many women athletes now wish to continue their physical training during pregnancy. Recent research suggests there is no compelling reason why they should not do so. Indeed, the balance of evidence is in favour of exercise in uncomplicated pregnancies, with benefits for both mother and fetus. The evidence is provided in studies where physiological measures have been recorded at rest and during exercise throughout the course of a normal pregnancy.

Physiological responses to exercise were examined at low, moderate, and high exercise intensities in 10 pregnant women at each trimester. The heart rate and metabolic responses (oxygen consumption, ventilation) were compared to those in control subjects. The exercise chosen was stepping onto a bench for 5 min at each exercise level, with the intensity being increased by speeding up the rate of stepping. At the highest exercise intensity, the pregnant subjects were able to exercise at heart rates in the region of 155–160 beats min^{-1} without undue discomfort, except for local muscular fatigue in the third trimester. At comparable heart rates, the control subjects were able to do more work, but there was no apparent deterioration in the fitness of the experimental subjects as pregnancy progressed. The higher metabolic responses compared to the control subjects were largely accounted for by the increased bodyweight and the physiological adjustments to pregnancy found at rest (Williams *et al.* 1988).

A woman's mental state may also vary during pregnancy and can be monitored using a standard mood-adjective checklist. As pregnancy progresses researchers have noted a general trend towards increased fatigue and friendliness but decreased vigour and activity. When reviewed alongside the physiological responses, these observations suggest that there is no compelling physiological reason for inactivity during pregnancy, and that psychological factors may be more responsible for the decline in habitual activity, which is usually associated with pregnancy.

It is now acknowledged that exercise should be promoted in healthy individuals with uncomplicated pregnancies. Clearly, some activities are unsuitable and exercise in hot conditions should be avoided. Serious runners will need to curtail their training, if only because of the discomfort due to the alterations in gait and the extra body mass to be lifted against gravity. Warning signs include pain, bleeding, rupture of membranes, and absence of fetal movements.

Although it is hard to make individual prescriptions, many women do manage to restore their training to moderate levels soon after delivery. Both Mary Slaney and Ingrid Kristensen returned to training within 1 week of giving birth. Liz McColgan gained a medal in the World Cross-Country Championships 5 months after giving birth to her first daughter and 4 months later won the world title on the track over 10,000 m. It is, of course, difficult to return to serious training due to disrupted sleep patterns, extra hydration needs for lactation, and so on. Despite these difficulties, there are many examples of women returning to serious competition within 6 months of giving birth and some produce career-best performances once their family has been started. Indeed, there may be a residual effect of hCG, a hormone secreted profusely during pregnancy, which benefits exercise performance after the baby's birth.

9.9 Overview

We have reached the stage where many myths about the limited capabilities of the female athlete have been overturned, particularly with regard to restraints on exercise performance. A female athlete shows similar physiological adaptations to training as do males but may be vulnerable to athletic anaemia, particularly if dietary iron intake is inadequate. The feats performed by today's top women runners would have been unthinkable two decades ago. Pioneers like Grete Waitz and her compatriot, Ingrid Kristensen, and a host of British, continental European, and American women have been responsible for pushing back the frontiers in women's long-distance racing. These have been further extended by the outstanding performances by Chinese distance runners in the 1993 competitive season and the increasing (albeit still small) number of adult African runners now training seriously. **They are reflected also in the popularity of women's running and its relative safety for them,** and by the rapid growth in women participating in soccer and rugby. The sports-clothing industry has responded to this burgeoning market by designing footwear for women rather than offering modified men's wear. Similarly runners' clothing – shoes, vests and sports bras – are now freely available, and are designed to fit the female form with comfort and efficiency.

The tremendous thrusts in the sports performance of elite women athletes have demonstrated interactions with the normal menstrual cycle. Some sports, notably gymnastics and ballet, are associated with a delayed menarche. Secondary amenorrhea is linked with impairment of the hypothalamic–pituitary–gonadal axis in highly competitive endurance athletes. A further related problem is reduced bone mineral density when amenorrhea persists for a prolonged period and is linked to the resulting low levels of oestrogen. Performance is limited but is not necessarily restricted during pregnancy.

Further reading

Puhl, J. L. and Brown, C. H. (1986) *The menstrual cycle and physical activity*. Human Kinetics, Champaign, Illinois.

Shangold, M. (1985). *Exercise and the female*. Academic Press, New York.

References

Bonen A., Belcastro, A.N., Ling, W.Y., and Simpson, A.A. (1981). Profiles of selected hormones during menstrual cycles of teenage athletes. *J. Appl. Physiol.*, **50**, 545–51.

Dalton, K. (1978). *Once a month*. Fontana, London.

De Mendoza, S. G. Nuceta, H. J., Salazar, E., Zerpa, A., and Kashyap, M. L. (1979). Plasma lipids and lipoprotein lipase activator property during the menstrual cycle. *Horm. Metabol. Res.*, **11**, 696–7.

Drinkwater, B. L. (1986). Female endurance athletes. Human Kinetics, Champaign. Illinois, USA.

Drinkwater, B. (1988). Training of female athletes. In The Olympic book of sports medicine (ed. A. Dirix, H. G. Knuttgen, and K. Tittel), pp.309–27. Blackwell, Oxford.

Hackney, A. C., McClacken-Compton, M. A., and Ainsworth, B. (1994). Substrate responses to submaximal evidence in the midfollicular and midluteal phases of the menstrual cycle. *Int. J. Sports Nutr.*, **4**, 299–308.

Higdon, H. (1981). Running through pregnancy. *The Runner*, December, 46–51.

Jurowski-Hall, J. E., Jones, M. L., Trews, C. J., and Sutton, J. R. (1981). Effects of menstrual cycle on blood lactate, oxygen delivery and performance during exercise. *J. Appl. Physiol.*, **51**, 1493–9.

Marker, K. (1981). Influence of athletic training on the maturity process of girls. *Medicine Sport*, **15**, 117–26.

Möller-Nielsen, J. and Hammar, M. (1989). Women's soccer injuries in relation to the menstrual cycle and oral contraceptive use. *Med. Sci. Sports Exerc.*, **21**, 126–9.

O'Reilly, A. and Reilly, T. (1990). Effects of the menstrual cycle and response to exercise. In *Contemporary ergonomics 90* (ed. E. J. Lovesey), pp. 149–3. Taylor and Francis, London.

Phillips, S. K., Rook, K. M., Siddle, N. C., Bruce, S. A., and Woledge, R. C. (1993). Muscle weakness in women occurs at an earlier age than in men, but strength is preserved by hormonal replacement therapy. *Clin. Sci.*, **84**, 95–8.

Reilly, T. and Rothwell, J. (1988). Adverse effects of overtraining in females. In *Contemporary ergonomics 88* (ed. E. D. Megaw), pp. 316–21. Taylor and Francis, London.

Warren, M. P. (1980). The effects of exercise on pubertal progression and reproductive function in girls. *J. Clin. Endocrinol. Metabol.*, **51**, 1150–6.

Williams, A., Reilly, T., Campbell, I., and Sutherst, J. (1988). Investigation of changes in response to exercise and in mood during pregnancy. *Ergonomics*, **31**, 1539–49.

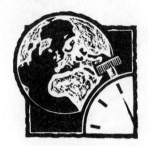

10
Seasonal variations

10.1 Introduction

Throughout the chapters of this textbook on biological rhythms, a spectrum of rhythm periods has been examined, ranging from the ultradian stages of sleep, through the circadian fluctuations in physiological and performance variables, to the infradian rhythm of the menstrual cycle. In this chapter, biological rhythms with even longer periods than the circamensal cycle are examined – those that recur once per year. Such rhythms may be defined as 'circannual', which denotes a period of about 1 year $\pm$ 2 months, or 'seasonal'. Strictly speaking, seasonal changes are brought about by changes in environmental fluctuations and are not observed in the absence of such changes, whereas circannual rhythms may be endogenous and/or desynchronized from the calendar year. The variations over the year that are considered in this chapter will be termed 'seasonal', since it is often not known in humans whether a particular circannual rhythm is endogenous or exogenous in origin. In this chapter, we examine seasonal variations in the habitual levels of leisure-time physical activity, physical fitness, and competitive sports performance. The possible mechanisms behind why the symptoms of some psychological disorders show significant seasonal changes are also discussed.

10.2 Seasonal rhythms – influences and mechanisms

10.2.1 The earth's seasons

All regions of the earth show marked seasonal variation, except those at, or very close to, the Equator. Seasons are caused by the elliptical orbit of the earth around the sun and the axis of the daily rotation of the earth being inclined at 23.5° from the vertical. These two astronomical characteristics have the effect of producing variation in both the duration of daylight and the angle at which the rays of the sun strike the surface of the Earth. These phenomena combine to cause a seasonal variation in climate.

There are many different climates on earth, with most varying to some degree with the time of year. As one moves, in either direction away from the tropical, forested equatorial regions, one travels through the subtropical belt of hot deserts, then through a temperate region of mild winters and cool summers to, eventually, the polar regions of extremely cold winters and 'summers', which are still just a few degrees above 0° C. Generally, as one travels away from the equatorial regions, the climate becomes more seasonal and the length of daylight within a 24-hour period deviates from the constant 12 hours observed at the Equator. This is most apparent close to the Earth's poles. For example, the Norwegian town of Alta (latitude, 69° 58′ north; longitude, 23° 15′ east) experiences 24 hours of complete darkness for 2 months in the winter, but between the 18th of May and the 24th of July, the entire sun is above the horizon for 24 hours per day. A large seasonal variation in climate can also be found in temperate regions that are far from the sea (e.g. Moscow in Russia). The fact that such regions of the Earth are populated by, among others, athletes, illustrates the importance of considering the effects of seasonal variations in climate and length of day.

10.2.2 The importance of predicting seasonal changes

Seasonal cycles are essential for the survival of many species of animals and plants. The most obvious example is the timing of breeding so that young animals are born at an appropriate time of year (usually just prior to the season associated with an abundancy of food). Changes in fur pigmentation and growth, as well as animal behaviour (migration, hibernation) also occur cyclically over the course of a year. These changes are triggered by fluctuations in daylight, environmental temperature or, more rarely, the moon (the Pacific palolo worm spawns at dawn, exactly 1 week after the full moon in November). The most significant stimuli on animal reproduction and behaviour are the environmental influence of the length of day, and the mediating daylight-dependent hormone, melatonin, which is secreted from the pineal gland. Both these stimuli have been exploited in agriculture; for example, the production of eggs from hens, the number of lambs born per ewe in sheep, the growth of fur in mink, and the breeding of racehorses can now all be manipulated artificially using chronobiological techniques.

Unlike animals and plants, humans in modern societies can control both the temperature in their immediate surroundings and the amount of light they are exposed to within a 24-hour period. Consequently, the habitual activity and behaviour of humans are no longer tightly bound to seasonal fluctuations in the length of day as they have been for thousands of years. This is well-illustrated by ancient monuments, such as Stonehenge in England or New Grange in Ireland, which are aligned with the sun in order to recognize the time of year. Nevertheless, seasonal rhythms are still evident in humans, though, as already stated, it is more difficult than with animals to establish the relative endogenous and exogenous influences on these rhythms. For example, human birth-rates vary with the time of year, but are tightly linked to environmental cycles only in populations living near to the Earth's poles (e.g. the Inuits and Eskimos). In developed countries, seasonal variations in human behaviour and activity (and therefore physical fitness and health) are greatly affected by cultural, religious and economic influences (see below). Even if these factors are controlled, there still remains the problem of studying human subjects for long periods of time, whether in temporal isolation (if the endogeneity of the rhythm is to be established) or merely during their everyday lives. Humans *have* spent more than 1 year in isolation units, but, strictly speaking, much more than one cycle of a rhythm should be examined to define any rhythm characteristics accurately. Together with the rigorous control that is required for 12 months or more, the interactions of rhythms of different periods have to be considered in order to characterize a seasonal variation reliably. For example, sampling at the same time of day for many days would not take into account any seasonal rhythms in circadian amplitudes, which have been documented with, for example, body temperature. Research into seasonal rhythms is presently at a similar stage to that in circadian rhythms 40 years ago; evidence suggests that human seasonal rhythms are, in part, endogenously mediated, but until adequate measurement protocols which control all exogenous influences are devised, it is hard to prove this undeniably. Despite the present methodological problems, some tentative conclusions can be made regarding the mechanisms of human seasonal rhythms.

10.3 Seasonal changes in the human

10.3.1 Birth-rates

Since the most significant seasonal effects are evident in the reproductive behaviour of animals, it is of interest to examine whether such rhythms exist in humans. In the USA and Europe, human sexual activity, the incidence of rapes and sexual transmitted diseases, as well as sales of contraceptives, all peak towards the end of the summer at the same time that plasma levels of the sex hormone testosterone reach a seasonal maximum (Smolensky 1992). It is impossible to implicate this hormone as an endogenous mechanism, since many factors may mediate these sexual cycles. For example, summer is the peak-time for holidays during which social contacts may increase. Besides, other sexual cycles related to birth-rates (e.g. sperm count) are *lowest* in the summer months.

There may be a bias for elite athletes to be born in September and October. This is more likely to be due to developmental and sociological reasons than, as has been claimed, "biorhythms". Children born at these times of year would be the oldest in their school years and, hence, at a more advanced stage developmentally. Given the rapid increases in strength and endurance after, compared to before, puberty, the oldest children in a school year of 13–14 year-olds would be more likely to be successful at school sport. This may, in turn, increase the chances of their receiving specialized coaching and continuing with sport into adulthood.

10.3.2 Levels of physical activity and physical fitness in the general population

The greatest seasonality in behaviour is found in animals living close to the poles. Consequently, humans living in such regions might be expected to decrease their activity levels markedly in the winter period of continuous darkness. Those Canadian Eskimos who still live a hunter–gatherer existence do *not* seem to 'hibernate' in winter (Shephard 1978). Conversely, they continue to hunt mammals and fish, expending significant amounts of energy. It is apparent, however, that acculturated Eskimos and other employed people who live in polar regions do reduce their levels of physical activity in the winter. For example, Wedahl (1990) found that the levels of sport participation in subjects living in Norway (measured as the sum of duration and perceived exertion in each activity) mirrored the seasonal changes in daylight hours. Such fluctuations in physical activity levels probably mediate corresponding changes in physical fitness. Erikssen and Rodahl (1979) examined 1835 Norwegian men and found that performances in 'a near-maximal bicycle test' were significantly better in summer than in winter. Ingleman-Hansen and Halkjaer-Kristensen (1982) also reported that the VO_2 *max* of Danish soldiers was significantly higher in summer than in winter.

At lower latitudes, levels of activity are still generally higher than in the summer. Dannenberg *et al.* (1989) examined the seasonal variation in physical activity in subjects living in New England, USA. Walking for pleasure was the most frequent activity for men in spring and summer and for women in all four seasons. As expected, activities like skiing increased in the winter, while swimming and gardening increased in the summer. Ignoring the type of activity, the subjects were again more active in the summer than the winter, in terms of the number of activities, duration of activity, and energy expended. However, the participation of 'conditioning' activities (those involving an energy expenditure of at least 31.4 kJ min^{-1}) did not show a seasonal variation. Such a maintenance in activity levels all year round may be important for decreasing the risk of acute coronary events. Although, in the general population, the incidences of myocardial infarctions and strokes peak in winter, an abrupt initiation of intense exercise in the summer after a winter period of detraining may be dangerous. Uitenbroek (1993) examined the seasonal variation in leisure-time physical activity in Scottish subjects. Independent of the level or type of activity, less people participated in sports in the winter compared to summer, with the changes throughout the year showing a sinusoidal pattern (Fig. 10.1). It was also found in this study that the times for most activities peaked later in the year (at the end of summer) for subjects aged 46–60 years. The winter reduction in activity appeared to be unrelated to the cessation of exercise altogether.

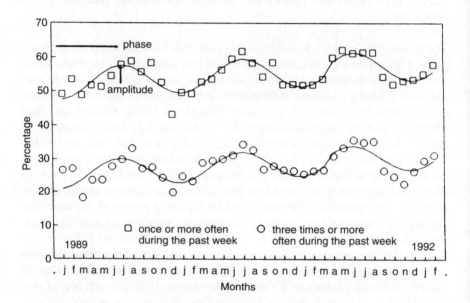

Fig. 10.1 Percentage of Scottish subjects participating in leisure sport throughout the year (Uitenbroek, 1993).

Although probably the above seasonal variations in physical fitness are exogenously mediated by levels of activity, it is unclear whether the latter changes are governed, in such extreme latitudes, by increases in the number of daylight hours or more favourable environmental temperatures. Besides, there are several other influences on seasonal variations in physical fitness. In fact, it is extremely difficult to generalize on the mechanisms behind seasonal variations in the types and levels of activity carried out by human subjects living in nonpolar regions. This is illustrated by a study carried out by Cumming and Bailey (1974) on Canadian farmers. The maximal oxygen uptake of these subjects was 10% higher at the end of winter compared to the end of summer. Body fat was also lower in the winter, even though the farmers carried out harvesting work in the summer. The authors attributed these findings to increased mechanization of farming methods and the fact that the subjects participated in the winter sport of curling. Kwarecki *et al.* (1981) also found a peak in physical fitness at the start of spring in Polish subjects, although another peak in fitness was observed in August. These authors examined a more heterogeneous group of subjects in terms of the type of sports participation (winter or summer). These findings suggest that the strongest influence on seasonal changes in physical fitness are no longer seasonal changes in the amount of occupational work, but rather fluctuations over 12 months in the amount of activity carried out in leisure-time.

10.3.3 Competitive sports performance

Seasonal changes in climate have undoubtedly influenced the development of sport and behaviour of elite athletes. Activities such as cricket are designated appropriate for the warmer summer temperatures, whereas robust field games are contested in the winter. The so-called 'winter sports' incorporated into the winter Olympics are performed on snow or on ice. These include skiing, ice-skating, tobogganing and ski-jumping. Recently, the distinction between winter and summer sports has become blurred with the introduction of indoor facilities and the accessibility of travel across hemispheres to reverse seasons. Many athletes from the northern hemisphere continue high levels of training and competition in the winter by migrating to Australia or Florida. English cricket tours of India and Pakistan are also usually undertaken in December.

Seasonal variation in the performance of elite sports participants is difficult to detect against the background of random variation found in laboratory tests of physical fitness. White *et al.* (1982) examined seasonal changes in the anthropometric (e.g. body composition) and performance variables of the British road-race cycling squad. Several variables were observed to be 'better' in the competitive season (e.g. percentage body fat, $\dot{V}O_2$ max and anaerobic power). Reilly and Thomas (1977) employed the more appropriate multivariate analyses to assess changes in fitness components of footballers throughout the year. The most pronounced changes were linked to the preseason period of conditioning which followed a close-season lay-off. Throughout the competitive season, fitness measures remained relatively stable. Professional soccer players are released from training in the summer, after a hard competitive season, and conventionally choose to carry out minimal amounts of activity for 6–8 weeks. Fluctuations in fitness over a year may be harder to detect in athletes who remain relatively active outside their competitive season. Van Ingen Schenau *et al.* (1992) found that, despite an increase in both training volume and intensity in the competitive season, a sample of elite Dutch speed-skaters showed no seasonal variation in $\dot{V}O_2$ max and performance in the Wingate 30-second test of anaerobic power (Fig. 10.2). These authors also cited work that showed that seasonal changes in laboratory-measured $\dot{V}O_2$ max are not evident for American speed-skaters, elite swimmers and middle-distance runners. Similarly, seasonal fluctuations in $\dot{V}O_2$ max could not be detected for female basketball players (Crouse et al. 1992). In Chapter 4, it was stated that it is rare to detect circadian variation in $\dot{V}O_2$ max which seems to be a stable function. Performance in the Wingate test does not consistently show a circadian rhythm. The insensitivity of the tests mentioned in Chapter 4 may also mean that they cannot detect changes that occur with the time of year, especially within the competitive season, in athletes who are well-trained all year round.

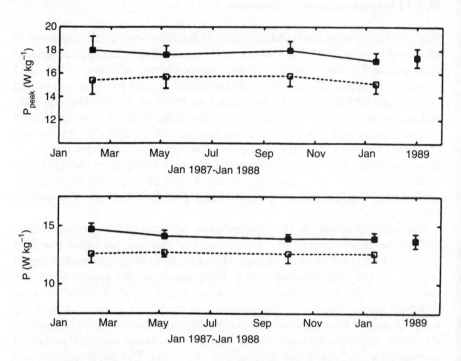

Fig. 10.1 Mean and peak power output in Dutch speed skaters. Mean ($\pm$SD) values are shown for men (filled symbols) and women (open symbols) – from Van Ingham Schenan *et al.* (1992).

Serious athletes conventionally 'periodize' or 'cycle' their training throughout the year. Periodization (not to be confused with the chronobiological definition of the period of a rhythm) is based on Selye's general adaptation syndrome and consists of cyclic variations in the intensity and types of training stimuli and the amount of rest. In sports such as American Football and professional soccer, considerable emphasis is placed on the preseason period of conditioning which usually lasts about 6 weeks. During this period, aerobic factors improve, but strength and anaerobic power may be compromised if they are neglected in the design of a training programme which emphasises endurance. In sprinting and middle-distance racing, athletes tend to improve during the competitive season by timing the quantity of speed training to achieve top performances in the major meetings. Where two or more major championships are included in the competitive season, training programmes are altered to achieve bimodal or multimodal intraseasonal cycles in fitness. While periodization techniques have been shown to be an effective method of training and should be related to seasonal variations in the level of competition, there is absolutely no scientific basis for linking periodization techniques to 'biorhythm theory' (e.g. resting on 'trough days' and training hard on 'crest days'). There have been anecdotal reports of improvements in athletic performance by altering the amount of training in response to whether a 'good day' or a 'bad day' was predicted, but these are probably the result of periodically resting a previously overtraining athlete. Similarly, there is no rationale for avoiding competition, if adequately prepared, on the basis of one's so-called 'biorhythms'.

10.3.4 Physiological variables

There is a large variation in the acrophases reported for seasonal rhythms in hormonal secretion, even in subjects living in the same climatic regions. For example, follicle-stimulating hormone has been found to peak in February and October (Nicolau and Haus 1989); plasma testosterone peaks in both winter (Nicolau and Haus 1989) and summer (Smolensky 1992); human growth hormone peaks in April; and cortisol and insulin peak in winter. Such large differences in the timing of seasonal endocrine rhythms suggest that these cycles are more influenced by exogenous (e.g. environmental temperature changes) than by endogenous mechanisms. Physical exercise may be a significant mediating factor; the changes during a season in the levels of plasma testosterone and cortisol in elite female rowers mirror closely the changes in training volume (Vervoorn *et al.* 1992).

Systolic and diastolic blood pressures are higher in winter than in summer, though the differences are probably due to changes in environmental temperature rather than any endogenous rhythm. In corroboration, peak incidences of myocardial infarctions and thrombotic strokes occur in winter. Other measures related to cardiovascular disease, which are higher in winter compared to summer, are plasma concentrations of total lipids and cholesterol.

It is not clear to what extent (if at all) seasonal changes in physiological measures influence fitness factors independently of the training and competitive regimes employed. Longer hours of daylight in the summer mean that the synthesis of vitamin D is increased. This fat-soluble vitamin promotes the growth and mineralization of bones and increases the absorption of dietary calcium. The density of bone mineral is least in the winter months, but it is difficult to conclude that this is due to vitamin D depletion since physical activity levels are also minimal at this time of year (Bergstralh *et al.* 1990). Besides, there are only small differences in athletes' diets between the competitive season and the off-season (*Nutter* 1991).

There is a three-week cycle in the remodelling of bone. Osteoclasts, which absorb bone, exist in small masses within bone. Over a period of 3 weeks, these collections of osteoclasts can absorb 'tunnels' of bone that may be as great as 1 mm in diameter and several mm in length. Bone deposition then occurs for several months until the tunnel is filled. It is not known whether the action of such conglomerates of osteoclasts is synchronized, which would result every few weeks in a cycle in bone mineral density.

Sweating during exercise occurs earlier after the onset of exercise and more profusely in summer than in winter, while the sodium concentration of sweat is less in the summer. It appears that these seasonal differences are mediated by the degree of acclimatization to warmer temperatures, since, when subjects are prewarmed for 30 min at 30 °C in the winter, sweating characteristics are no different from those in the summer. During the summer, it could be argued that warmer environmental temperatures encourage athletes to work at higher training stimuli than in the winter, mediating greater training adaptations. This may depend on the duration of exercise since precooling body temperature (an effect which a cool season may simulate) increases work-rates during prolonged exercise, such as marathon running.

One variable that varies seasonally and may not be totally dependent on activity levels is the amount of adipose tissue in the body. Zahorska-Markiewicz and Markiewicz (1984) discovered that body fat was highest in the summer months, even though the physiological responses to exercise at an intensity of 60 W indicated that the subjects were fitter at this time. These researchers noted that RER during exercise was higher in the summer, indicating that relatively less fatty acids were being used as fuel. This agrees with the fact that basal metabolism is higher in winter and spring than in summer and autumn.

10.4 Human pineal function

In animals, the pineal gland mediates the transmission of environmental light/dark information to physiological systems through the secretion of melatonin. Removal of the gland destroys the ability of animals to measure the length of day, and although seasonal rhythms persist, they are desynchronized from the environment. Therefore, the pineal gland appears to communicate zeitgeber information to an underlying endogenous annual rhythm of seasonality (Arendt 1992). Although the significance of the effects of melatonin in humans is unresolved, humans show an unequivocal and marked daylight-dependent rhythm in melatonin secretion. Melatonin production from its precursors, tryptophan and serotonin, occurs mainly at night in a normal environment (Fig. 10.3). Plasma concentrations begin to rise at about 21:00 to a maximum between 01:00 and 05:00. There is considerable interindividual differences in the amplitude of this circadian rhythm.

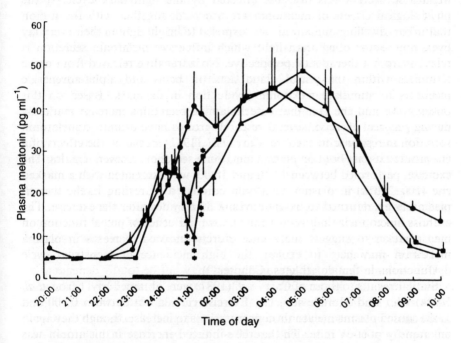

Fig. 10.3 The effect of light on the nocturnal secretion of melatonin (Drendt, 1992): a – dim light; b – light of 300 lux; c – light of 2500 lux.

The melatonin rhythm is phase-advanced in summer compared to winter and there may be a small increase in duration of the nocturnal secretion in winter. Early attempts to manipulate the rhythm in melatonin experimentally with artificial light were unsuccessful due to the use of low intensities of light. Apparently, the light required to suppress melatonin secretion in humans is far brighter (>2500 lx) than that used successfully in animal studies (Fig. 10.3). This means that domestic intensities of light (about 500 lx) cannot reproduce the effects on melatonin of natural light (>10,000 lx). Thus, the consideration of any physiological effects of melatonin secretion (or the lack of it) is important for people who are rarely exposed to natural daylight (e.g. blind athletes). Therapeutic possibilities of bright light and exogenous melatonin have been suggested for the treatment of disturbances to circadian rhythms caused by shiftwork and time-zone transitions (Chapters 6–8). The main implication of the human pineal gland for seasonal rhythms is in the relationship between it and the incidence of certain affective disorders.

10.4.1 Effects of exercise on melatonin secretion

Melatonin secretion is not just affected by the light–dark cycle. If the physiological effects of melatonin are accepted, together with the notion that urban-dwelling humans are less exposed to bright light in their everyday lives, any factor other than light which influences melatonin secretion is relevant from a therapeutic perspective. Noradrenaline released from nerve terminals within the pineal gland acts on beta- and alpha-adrenergic receptors to stimulate melatonin production in the dark. Based on this observation and the fact that catecholamine secretions increase markedly during physical exercise, several research groups have examined melatonin secretion in response to exercise. Carr *et al.* (1981) measured the effects of a 60-minute exercise bout on plasma melatonin secretion in seven females. The exercise, performed between 13:00 and 18:00, was associated with a marked rise (100–200%) in plasma melatonin compared to resting levels, though plasma levels returned to baseline within 30 minutes after the exercise. The authors linked their findings with the known influence of pineal function on menstruation to suggest that acute exercise-induced increases in plasma melatonin may help to explain the high incidence of menstrual cycle dysfunctions in female athletes (Chapter 9).

Similar results to those of Carr *et al.* (1981) were obtained by Theron *et al.* (1984) who studied male subjects. Exercise carried out between 09:00 and 13:00 caused plasma melatonin concentrations to increase, though they again fell rapidly post-exercise. The exercise-induced increase in melatonin was even greater when subjects exercised in a dark room (54 lx). This suggests that the photoperiodic influence on melatonin is not reduced, but accentuated during exercise, although it is stressed that the exercise, whatever the light condition, was performed during the hours of environmental daylight. Montelone *et al.* (1990) exercised male subjects at 22:40 for 20 min and measured plasma melatonin concentrations nocturnally, before and after the exercise. The results clearly showed that, contrary to the previous work, the melatonin concentration was significantly lower than the control levels for 3 hours post-exercise (Fig. 10.4).

Despite the above conflicting results, it is clear that exercise does influence melatonin secretion to a degree that may depend on the timing of exercise within the solar day and/or the amount of exposure to light. Physical activity continued over the course of the year may have a prophylactic effect with respect to seasonal mood changes. Further work should examine the effects of exercise scheduling on melatonin secretion and should investigate whether exercise can, like bright light and exogenous melatonin, manipulate circadian rhythms and help alleviate the problems associated with seasonal affective disorder (SAD).

10.4.2 Seasonal patterns of affective-disorder symptoms

The seasonality of manic depression has been well documented since the original observations made by Hippocrates and Socrates suggested such a phenomenon. The peak incidences of clinical symptoms of all major depressive illnesses occur in spring and, to a lesser extent, in autumn. There

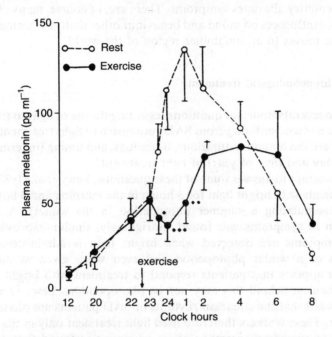

Fig. 10.4 The effects of nocturnal exercise on the secretion of melatonin (Montelone *et al.*, 1990)

is also indirect evidence which supports the timing of these peaks. For example, rates of depression-related suicide, the use of antidepressive drugs, and depression-diagnosed hospital admissions all peak in the spring and autumn.

Seasonal affective disorder, on the other hand, refers exclusively to depression that occurs in winter. The criteria for clinical diagnosis are that patients should be depressed for two successive winters without the presence of summer depression or social causality. Consequently, SAD is seasonally distinct from other forms of depression. The more common depressive symptoms of sadness, anxiety, lethargy, and poor concentration are present in SAD, but patients also report more unusual symptoms of carbohydrate craving, increased eating, and longer sleep-times. Consequently, patients with SAD have been described colloquially as 'hibernators'.

10.4.3 Relation to environmental light

The photoperiod is the interval between the first and last exposure to light each day. It is possible that SAD is a photoperiodic phenomenon; some patients with winter depression claim that their illness started on moving from a tropical to a temperate climate. Others report that a winter visit to a tropical country alleviates symptoms. There are, of course, many changes in exogenous influences on mood and behaviour other than environmental light when one moves to an unfamiliar region of the world.

10.4.4 Chronobiological treatment

There are several important questions regarding the use of light to treat SAD. First, are humans suffering from SAD responsive to light treatment at all? If so, what are the optimum durations, intensities, and timing (in terms of both time of day and time of year) of light treatment?

In an attempt to answer some of these questions, Lewy *et al.* (1982) treated SAD patients with bright light for 3 hours in the morning and 3 hours in the evening (simulating a summer photoperiod in the winter). A dramatic remission in symptoms was found. Intriguingly, similar improvements in SAD symptoms are observed when bright light is administered at the extremes of a winter photoperiod and even when given at midday. It therefore appears that patients respond to treatment with bright light but the mechanism behind this may not be photoperiodic. Lewy *et al.* (1987) hypothesized that the circadian rhythms of SAD patients are phase-delayed in winter. These workers therefore used light treatment only in the morning in order to provide a corrective phase-advance and found that symptoms dramatically improved. Again, there can be dramatic improvements in SAD symptoms without such timing of light treatment. It is, therefore, apparent that there are reasons to support SAD being a photoperiodic phenomenon, though the success of phototherapy does not seem to depend on the photoperiodic timing of treatment.

10.5 Climatic events

Seasonal climatic changes can mediate fluctuations in negative and positive air-ions. The break-up of water droplets, such as occurs during a rainy season, increases the concentration of negative-ions in the air, whereas the movement of large volumes of air over a land mass may increase positive air-ions. The latter phenomenon gained the attention of sports scientists prior to the 1972 Munich Olympics when there was concern that the Foehn wind from Central Europe towards the south of Germany might adversely affect the performance of athletes. Positive-ions have been correlated with negative mood-states. Negative-ions are thought to promote improvements in mood, hence the commercial availability of negative air-ion generators which can be placed in the home or office. Although air-ions have been found to be biologically active, influencing serotonin levels, body temperature, and metabolism, these effects tend to diminish under strenuous exercise conditions (Reilly 1990).

The rest–activity cycle is biannually adjusted by 1 hour in many temperate countries. Clocks are adjusted forward in the spring and backwards in the autumn. Since little change has occurred in the timing of the light–dark cycle, circadian rhythms may take several days to entrain back to clock-time. During this period of competing zeitgebers, psychomotor performance deteriorates (Reilly 1990). Whether sports performance is detrimentally affected during this time is not known.

10.6 Overview

In the general population of the northern hemisphere, habitual levels of physical activity and physical fitness are higher in the summer than in the winter. Although partly influenced by the photoperiod, these variations should be considered as 'seasonal' rather than 'circannual', since it is unclear whether winter reductions in physical activity are mediated by the decreased hours of daylight, giving less opportunity for sport or melatonin-influenced changes in mood in the winter. For most people, the increasingly sedentary nature of occupational tasks means that physical activity in leisure-time has the strongest influence on variations in physical fitness. Consequently, athletes engaged in winter sports are probably fitter at this time of year. It is difficult, however, to identify seasonal variations in $\dot{V}O_2$ max and other laboratory tests of exercise performance with well-trained athletes, despite obvious changes in their competitive performances throughout the year. This can be attributed to the relative lack of measurement sensitivity in laboratory indices of performance, together with the fact that athletes remain active, even out of their competitive seasons. Most seasonal changes in physiological measures are related to lower environmental temperatures in the winter. In very inactive individuals, the higher basal metabolic rate in winter may mean that body fat is less during this season than in summer. In athletes, seasonal physiological changes reflect the amount of training that is performed. There are circadian and seasonal rhythms in melatonin secretion in humans which are mediated by the light–dark cycle. Bright light and exogenous melatonin are now being examined with respect to their use in coping with rhythm disturbances and SAD. Physical exercise also affects melatonin secretion, supporting the hypothesis that it is a significant zeitgeber in humans. More work is needed to establish the exact relationships between bright light, physical activity, and melatonin secretion, as well as the effects of melatonin on seasonal and circadian rhythms.

Further reading

Van Ingen Schenau, G. J., Bakker, F. C., de Groot, G., and de Koning, J. J. (1992). Supramaximal cycle tests do not detect seasonal progression in performance in groups of elite speed skaters. Europ. J. Appl. Physiol. Occupat. Physiol., 64, 292–7.

References

Arendt J. (1992). The pineal. In *Biological rhythms in clinical and laboratory medicine* (ed. Y. Touitou and E. Haus), pp. 348–62. Springer-Verlag, Berlin.

Bergstralh, E. J., Sinaki, M., Offord, K. P., Wahner, H. W., and Melton, III, L. J. (1990). Effect of season on physical activity score, back extensor, muscle strength and lumbar bone mineral density. *J. Bone Min. Res.*, 5, 371–7.

Carr, D. B. (1981). Plasma melatonin increases during exercise in women. *J. Clin. Endocrinol. Metabol.*, 53, 224–5.

Crouse, S. F., Rohack, J. J., and Jacobsen, D. J. (1992). Cardiac structure and function in women basketball athletes: seasonal variation and comparisons with nonathletic controls. *Res. Quart. Exerc. Sport*, 63, 393–401.

Cumming, G. R., and Bailey, G. (1974). Seasonal variation of cardiorespiratory fitness of grain farmers. *J. Occupat. Med.*, 16, 91–3.

Dannenberg, A. L., Keller, J. B., Wilson, P. W. F., and Castelli, W. P. (1989). Leisure time physical activity in the Framingham Offspring study. *Am. J. Epidemiol.* 129, 76–88.

Erikssen, J. and Rodahl, K. (1979). Seasonal variation in work performance and heart rate responses to exercise. A study of 1,835 middle-aged men. *Europ. J. Appl. Physiol.*, 42, 133–40.

Ingleman-Hansen, T. and Halkjaer-Kristensen, J. (1982). Seasonal variation of maximal oxygen consumption rate in humans. *Europ. J. Appl. Physiol.*, 49, 151–7.

Kwarecki, K., Golec, L., Klossowski, M., and Zuzewicz, K. (1981). Circannual rhythms of physical fitness and tolerance of hypoxic hypoxia. *Acta Physiol. Pol.*, 32, 629–36.

Lewy, A. J., Kern, H. A., Rosenthal, N. E., and Wehr, T. A. (1982). Bright artificial light treatment of a manic depressive patient with a seasonal mood cycle. *Am. J. Psychiat.*, 139, 1496–8.

Lewy, A. J, Sack, R. L., Singer, C. M., and White, D. M. (1987). The phase-shift hypothesis for bright light's therapeutic mechanism of action. Theoretical considerations and experimental evidence. *Psychopharmacol. Bull.*, **23**, 349–53.

Monteleone, P., Maj, M., Fusco, M., Orazzo, C. and Kemali, D. (1990). Physical exercise at night blunts the nocturnal increase of plasma melatonin levels in healthy humans. *Life Sci.*, **47**, 1989–995.

Nicolau, G. Y. and Haus, E. (1989). Chronobiology of the endocrine system. *Rev. Roum. Med. Endocrinol.*, **27**, 153–83.

Nutter, J. (1991). Seasonal changes in female athletes diets. *Int. J. Sports Nutri.*, **1**, 395–407.

Reilly, T. (1990). Human circadian rhythms and exercise. *Crit. Rev. Biomed. Engin.*, **18**, 165–80.

Reilly, T. and Thomas, V. (1977). Application of multivariate analysis to the fitness assessment of soccer players. *Brit. J. Sports Med.*, **11**, 183–4.

Shephard, R. J. (1978). *Human physiological work capacity.* Cambridge University Press, Cambridge.

Smolensky, M. H. (1992). Chronoepidemiology: chronobiology and epidemiology. In *Biological rhythms in clinical and laboratory medicine* (ed. Y. Touitou and E. Haus), pp. 659–72. *Springer-Verlag, Berlin.*

Theron, J. J., Oosthuizen, J. M. C., and Rautenbach, M. M. (1984). Effect of physical exercise on plasma melatonin levels in normal volunteers. *S. Afri. Med. J.*, **66**, 838–41.

Uitenbroek D. G. (1993). Seasonal variation in leisure time physical activity. *Med. Sci. Sports Exerc*, **25**, 755–60.

Vervoorn, C., Vermulst, L. J. M., Boelens-Quist, A. M., Koppeschaar, H. P. F., Erich, W. B. M., Thijssen, J. H. H., and de Vries, W. R. (1992). Seasonal changes in performance and free testosterone: cortisol ratio of female elite rowers. *Europ. J. Appl. Physiol.*, **64**, 14–21.

Wedahl, A. (1990). Covariance of daylight, sport participation and sleep patterns. *Progr. Clin. Biol. Res.*, **341B**, 79–87.

White, J. A., Quinn, G., Al-Dawalibi, M., and Mulhall, J. (1982) Seasonal changes in cyclists' performance. Part I. The British Olympic road race squad. *Brit. J. Sports Med.*, **16**, 4–12.

Zahorska-Markiewicz, B. and Markiewicz, A. (1984). Circannual rhythm of exercise metabolic rate in humans. *Europ. J. Appl. Physiol.*, **52**, 328–30.

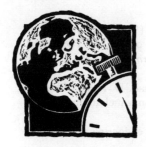

11
Research

In this book we have attempted to summarize what is known about rhythms and physical performance. It is clear that many questions remain to be answered and such answers will require well-designed experiments to be performed. Are there any special guidelines that apply to such experiments? This chapter represents a collation of advice and recommendations for the conduct of these studies.

11.1 Collecting data

All research workers want more data – but the case for this is stronger in the study of rhythms than in many other fields of research. If we are to study and characterize rhythms fully, intuitively we feel the need to collect data as frequently as possible over at least the period of the rhythm. Is this intuition correct and, if so, how frequently must we collect data?

11.1.1 Frequency of sampling

Constraints imposed by finance, time and ethics may limit the number of experiments. A restriction in the frequency of sampling can influence considerably the inference that can be drawn from a set of results. Consider, for example, Fig. 11.1. Fig 11.1a shows the concentration of plasma cortisol recorded at 30-minute, intervals during a single 24-hour period. Parts of these data are then replotted in Figures 11.1b–f, to show what would have been recorded with less frequent sampling. With hourly sampling (Fig. 11.1b), short-lived peaks or pulses are lost (e.g. as found in the first part of sleep) and, with 2-hour sampling (Figs. 1.11 c, d), only the major peaks are present. With 4-hour sampling (Figs. 11.1 e,f), only the general nature of the rhythm is preserved; the number and size of peaks and their timing can be described only approximately.

An analysis of urinary cortisol effectively provides an integrated sample (the mean of values since the last collection time); Fig. 11.1 g shows the results obtained when samples are collected every 2 h. In practice, urine sampling is often less frequent, with only a single overnight sample collected on rising (Fig. 11.1h). While an early morning sample gives information

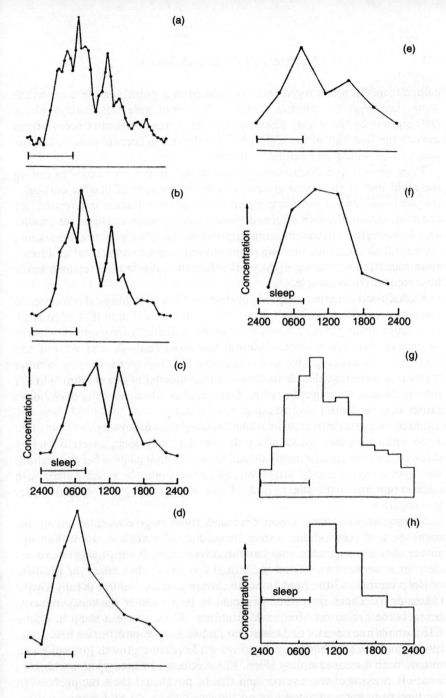

Fig. 11.1 Circadian rhythm of plasma cortisol (based on Krieger 1979), showing its shape when: (a) plotted half-hourly; (b) hourly; (c) 2-hourly at even hours; (d) 2-hourly at odd hours; (e) 4-hourly starting at 2400; (f) 4-hourly starting at 0200; (g) integrated two-hourly samples; (h) integrated 4-hourly samples and single overnight sample (Minors and Waterhouse 1988).

gained from the whole night and so differs from a 'point' sample taken at the same time (e.g. the plasma cortisol), it cannot give information about changes during the night. The fact that the lowest cortisol concentrations were in the first half of the night and that the rise in cortisol occurred in the second half would be completely missed.

Thus, when rapid fluctuations in concentration are expected – as during the night and in the hours around waking in the case of plasma cortisol – frequent sampling is most important if an accurate picture is required. By contrast, during the late afternoon and evening, when changes are smaller and less erratic, infrequent sampling is less likely to produce misleading results. Of course, if the phasing of the rhythm is not known, as after a time–zone transition or during night-work, then the experimenter cannot know how frequently to sample.

As discussed in earlier chapters, in studies of the physiological responses to exercise, most circadian rhythms are more symmetrical than that of cortisol. In practice, testing every 3 hours is generally sufficiently frequent for there to be enough data for a worthwhile mathematical analysis, and yet not too frequent to be unacceptable to the subjects. It is also worth bearing in mind that it is sometimes valuable to show the reproducibility of a rhythm. Thus, a total of 24 samples might be better distributed as 3-hour samples over 3 days rather than as 1-hour samples over only 1 day.

Three problems still remain when devising such experiments:

1. In order to assess rhythmicity due to the bodyclock, external factors (lifestyle and the environment) should be as constant as possible throughout the experimental periods. Moreover, all subjects must be synchronized with each other and with the period of the rhythms (e.g. 24 hours) under investigation.

2. Testing subjects every 3 hours requires them to give samples during the night. Should they remain awake throughout the night or be woken up? Either choice has its advantages and disadvantages. Staying awake increases sleep loss, whereas waking an individual avoids this, but raises the problem of sleep inertia and the need to make certain that the subject is fully awake (Chapter 5). These issues are particularly important if the measurements being taken are susceptible to such effects. Thus, whereas sleep has little effect on plasma cortisol and melatonin, it has a lowering effect on heart rate, blood pressure and body temperature, while plasma growth hormone and testosterone increased during sleep. These effects can take up to an hour to wear off. Staying awake avoids such effects, but then there is the problem of the negative effects of sleep loss on the subject's mood and mental performance.

3. Unlike with many other physiological variables, it is very difficult to administer a large number of consecutive performance tests to humans without eliciting fatigue. One solution to this problem is to have six test sessions spaced 4 hours apart within a 24-hour period at 02:00, 06:00, 10:00,

14:00, 18:00 and 22:00. Subjects are then divided so that they have their first test session at different times of the day. This protocol allows sufficient time for recovery after each test session and counterbalances any sequential effects that might occur. (By this is meant the possibility of a general decline (fatigue?) or rise (practice effect?) over the course of the six test sessions). As discussed above, there remain the problems associated with testing subjects during the night (at 02:00 and 06:00). To alleviate these problems, the experimental design can be modified so that at least 8 hours separate each of the six test sessions. The advantage of this protocol is that subjects can sleep normally between 22:00 and 06:00 on one test day and between 02:00 and 10:00 on the other.

4. With many performance variables, especially those of mental performance (Chapter 3) a practice effect may occur, in which, the performance improves with successive tests. The counterbalanced design described above also ameliorates this problem.

11.2 Analysing data

11.2.1 Combining and smoothing results

In nearly all experimental work, results are combined or averaged in some way. This might entail combining data from repeated samples from an individual, or pooling data from a group of subjects. A common example in chronobiology is to sample from different groups at different times during the 24-hour period. This is often the only way in which points covering the 24 hours can be obtained. However, such procedures are not without their problems when applied to studies of circadian rhythms. First, the different subjects must be in phase with one another, as has already been mentioned. This is generally achieved by exposing them to the same zeitgebers and standardizing their lifestyle. Failure to achieve such synchrony will tend to broaden the timing of any peaks and troughs and reduce the amplitude in grouped data. In the extreme situation of a completely desynchronized population, the combined output could be arrhythmic in spite of the individuals showing marked rhythms.

Second, the variable under consideration must show the same 24-hour mean and amplitude in the different subjects. Figure 11.2 shows the simple example of rhythms from three subjects (results from whom are indicated by curves a–c) that have the same amplitude and phase but different mean values. Each is sampled only at 6-hour intervals but, by staggering the sampling times for each subject by 2 hours, a 2-hour sampling frequency for the group as a whole is achieved. The shape of this grouped results bears no obvious relationship to those of the individuals; indeed the experimenter would be likely to draw the inference that an ultradian rhythm with a period of about 6 h was present in the results. This artefact will not be produced if the means (and amplitudes and phases) can be standardized in some way. Differences in mean values can be corrected for by expressing all values as a percentage of the 24-hour mean for that subject. Differences in amplitude are also corrected to some extent by this method but an alternative is to express results after z-transformation of the data. Finally, phases can be standardized by referring them to midsleep, or some other event which is known to affect phase, such as meal-times.

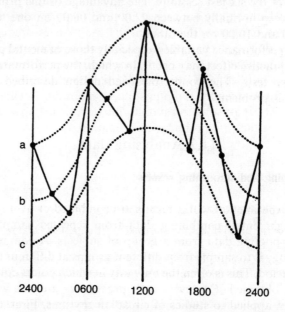

Fig. 11.2 Three sets of circadian data (a–c) with the same shape and amplitude but different means. The full line is the result of sampling from them sequentially. Further details are given in the text. (Minors and Waterhouse 1988.)

A method that is useful for showing general trends in data rather than rapid fluctuations is one which 'smoothes out' the differences between adjacent time-points by combining them in some way. In effect, this is automatically achieved with integrated samples (see above). Available techniques use weighted or unweighted means and combine different numbers of adjacent points. An unweighted three-point moving average requires calculating a value at time T_x which is the mean of values at T_{x-1}, T_x, T_{x+1}. An unweighted five-point moving average would use values obtained at times T_{x-2}, T_{x-1}, ... and T_{x+2}, and so on. Note that the number of calculated points decreases when the data are treated in this way, because moving averages cannot be calculated for the first and last time(s) of the original data-span. When a weighted three-point moving average is calculated, the central value of each set of three is emphasized, often in a ratio of 1:2:1. With a five-point moving average, the weightings might be 1:2:3:2:1. Note that such methods are inappropriate if the sampling points are unevenly spaced, that they tend to reduce the amplitude of the rhythm, and are of dubious value if samples are taken infrequently, say every 3 hours.

Smoothing the data in this way is not the same as decreasing the sampling frequency. Smoothing data or collecting integrated samples provides an averaged result that better describes a general trend at the expense of fluctuations, whether these are caused by hormonal secretory pulses, ultradian oscillations, or random fluctuations. By contrast, less frequent sampling of point data does not change the value that is measured at each time (Figs.11.1a–f). However, it does change the confidence with which a peak or trough can be identified, and increases the likelihood of missing such events because they fall between the sampling times. Smoothing is widely used when results are 'noisy', that is, when random fluctuations are large in relation to the amplitude of the rhythm under investigation.

11.2.2 Assessing rhythms with a 24-hour period

A rhythm can be described in terms of four parameters:

(1) the period or the time it takes for one cycle to be completed and for the pattern to repeat itself;
(2) the mean, or the average of all points within a single cycle;
(3) the amplitude, or the deviation of the peak and trough of the rhythm from its mean;
(4) the phase, or the timing of the rhythm with reference to some external standard, often expressed with respect to local midnight or midsleep.

Mathematical techniques exist for estimating these parameters (Minors and Waterhouse 1991), but the methods demand far longer spans of data and higher sampling frequencies when looking for the period of the data. These well-tried, tested methods, many of which were originally designed for use in the physical sciences, are beyond the scope of this article. The position is simplified if the period of the data is known or can be assumed, e.g. 24 h. In practice, this assumption can be made in studies performed upon subjects who have been living in a normal environment for at least several days previously. However, errors of interpretation will arise if this assumption is incorrect.

Assuming that any rhythmicity that is present has a period of 24 h, then two methods are commonly used to assess it. These are analysis of variance (ANOVA) and cosinor analysis.

11.2.2.1 Analysis of variance

A fairly simple method is a one-factor (time of day) analysis of variance (ANOVA). This assesses whether the variance between time-points is significantly greater than the random variation within them. The analysis requires several readings to be taken at each of a group of times within the day; the times of assessment do not have to be evenly spaced. The statistical tests are more likely to establish the presence of a time-of-day effect as the number of groups (time-points) and the number of values within each group increases. There are ANOVA tests that deal with replicated and unreplicated data, as well as with parametric and nonparametric measurements. (Strictly speaking, nonparametric tests are advised with data that have been 'standardized', as discussed above). Although it may be difficult to achieve in practice, a statistically powerful design is when the same subject is assessed at different times of day, because the replicated measurements remove inter-individual variation.

A strength of ANOVA methods is that the shape of the rhythm does not affect the statistical outcome. Thus, the sequence of time-points can be interchanged without statistical effect, even though the biological implication might be considerable. However, such an analysis, even if it established that rhythmicity exists, does not give information as to its shape, amplitude, mean, or phase. As only a few sampling times are taken, it is improbable that those corresponding to times of maximum and minimum would have been chosen, or that the mean of the samples would represent the true mean of the underlying rhythm.

11.2.2.2 Cosinor analysis

Cosinor analysis (Nelson *et al.* 1979) is probably the most enthusiastically promoted method for the analysis of rhythms, and statistical packages that deal with it are now available. It enables a set of data of a known period to be described in terms of its mesor (mean value of the fitted cosine curve), its amplitude, and its acrophase (time of peak of fitted curve).

Cosinor analysis is an objective assessment of all the data-span. In this respect, it has an advantage over methods which assess only maximum or minimum values, which are prone to the effects of a single aberrant value. From a statistical viewpoint, cosinor analysis simply investigates whether the data are better described by a cosine curve than by a straight line. A significant fit is taken as one for which the chance that the data are fitted as well by a horizontal line as by the cosine curve is less than 5 percent. (That is, it is one in which the amplitude of the fitted curve is significantly different from zero.) It is sometimes informative to assess the percentage of variability in the data that is accounted for by the fitted curve; this is the 'percentage rhythm'.

What assumptions does a cosinor analysis make, and what difficulties of interpretation exist with this method? First, the lack of a 'significant' fit does not indicate necessarily that no rhythm exists. Cosinor analysis is based on the major assumption that the data are approximately sinusoidal in shape. Obviously, this assumption is sometimes untrue. Rhythms with a shape closely approximating a cosine curve are uncommon. Examples include plasma phosphate on a constant diet and deep body temperature during free-running and constant routine conditions. Circadian rhythms vary greatly in their shape, which may be quite distinctive for a particular variable. The example of plasma cortisol has already been given (Fig. 11.1). A fairly common shape (Fig. 11.3*a*) is the 'saw-tooth' which rises steadily through the day and then falls more quickly during the night; blood urea nitrogen concentration approximates to this. Another fairly common shape is a 'square-wave' (Fig. 11.3*b*), in which two states or values alternate, for example the amount of activity during waking and sleep.

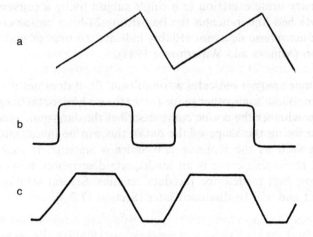

Fig. 11.3 Different shapes of circadian rhythm: (a) 'saw-tooth'; (b) square-wave; (c) 'ramp' function. In each case, two full cycles are shown Minors and Waterhouse 1988).

Given the wide variety in shapes of measured rhythms, one might legitimately question the validity of results obtained by cosinor analysis when the shape of the data differs from that of a perfect sinusoid. As the data-span departs from being sinusoidal in shape, the computed acrophase will be a less accurate indicator of the time of peak of the data, and the amplitude is an underestimate of the true value. These deviations are likely to be greater if the data are asymmetrical (e.g., Fig. 11.3*a*). In some cases (Fig. 11.4), the acrophase will be a poor measure of the time of 'peak', even though, in this case, the time of minimum will be more appropriate.

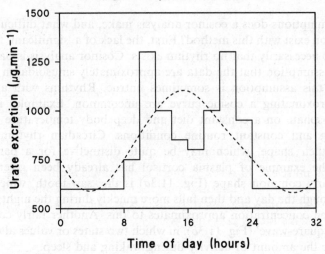

Fig. 11.4 Urinary urate excretion in a single subject living a conventional routine. The dashed line indicates the best-fitting 24-hour cosine curve. Note that the acrophase does not reliably indicate the time of maximal urate excretion (Minors and Waterhouse 1981).

Even if cosinor analysis indicates a 'significant' fit, it does not mean that the data do not follow some other shape (other than a horizontal line). If one wants to know whether the cosine curve describes the data-span adequately (here one is stressing the shape of the data), this can be investigated by a statistical test such as the Kolmogorov–Smirnov statistic. If such a test indicates that the cosine curve is an inadequate description, however, the problem of how best to describe the data remains. Several solutions have been suggested and will be discussed later (Section 11.2.4).

11.2.3 Interpreting changes in rhythm parameters as assessed by cosinor analysis

Often we wish to know if a rhythm has changed in response either to some experimental manipulation, e.g. a simulated time-zone transition. Interest often centres on the change in amplitude of the curve or the shift in its acrophase. Either result is associated with some interpretive problems that require comment.

11.2.3.1 Change of amplitude

If amplitude is lost to the extent that the cosine curve is no longer statistically significant, this implies that a cosine curve no longer fits the data-span better than a straight line. This is interesting in itself, of course, but there are several possible means of obtaining such a result, as summarized graphically in Figure 11.5. It is important to realize that rather different inferences can be drawn from each possibility and that visual inspection of the data will often help to distinguish between them. Thus, case 'a' implies that some mechanism is setting the variable at a maximum value (as would be the case with the effects of maximal sympathetic stimulation upon heart rate). Case 'd' is similar, except that there is a maximal inhibition (as might occur with resistance to blood flow in exercising muscles). In case 'b', there is the implication that the control rhythm was due to both increases and decreases about some tonic value. Finally, case 'c' implies the loss of some means of coordinating more rapid ultradian rhythms into a circadian whole.

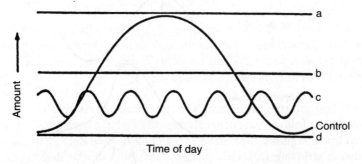

Fig. 11.5 Possible ways (a–d) in which circadian rhythmicity (control) can be lost. Further details are given in the text. (Minors and Waterhouse 1988).

If the experiment has been performed on pooled data, then the possibility of desynchronization exists and should be eliminated as a possible cause of the fall in amplitude (Section 11.2.1). For example, if the experimental manipulation removes zeitgebers and so prevents the internal clock from being synchronized, then individuals in a group will gradually lose their synchrony with each other. As a result, the combined rhythm will decrease in amplitude and become statistically nonsignificant. In these circumstances, the inspection of continuous data for each individual would show a rhythm of unchanged amplitude but with a slightly different free-running period. If the data have been obtained by pooling single samples from different individuals (e.g. Fig. 11.2), then there is no easy way to establish whether the subjects are arrhythmic, rather than rhythmic but asynchronous.

11.2.3.2 Change in acrophase

A change in acrophase cannot automatically be considered as an accurate measure of the amount by which a rhythm's phase has shifted. The shift in acrophase will be an accurate measure of the shift in rhythm only if the shapes of the two sets of data are the same. For example, Figure 11.6 shows sets of data which show acrophase changes, but only in the second example is the shift not produced by a change in shape.

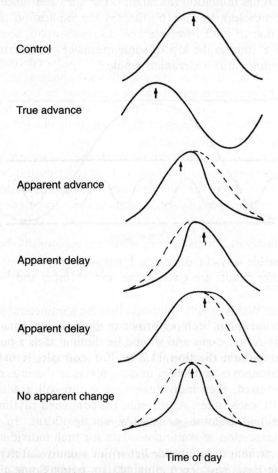

Fig. 11.6 Effect of changes in shape of data upon estimated acrophase, indicated by arrow (Minors and Waterhouse 1988).

There are three common reasons why a rhythm changes shape. The first is because the overt circadian rhythm is the sum of exogenous and endogenous components (Chapter 1). This means that following a change in lifestyle (e.g.

as occurs, after a time-zone transition), there may be a temporary loss of the normal matching between the two components. Thus, even though the shape of the components has not changed, that of the combination would have done so.

A second cause is a change in the shape of the exogenous component. This is possible because it is produced by the environment and behaviour (e.g. a change in training schedule). It is common in studies of shiftwork because dayworkers rest after working, but nightworkers generally take their leisure before they start their work. The results from a constant routine (Chapter 1) would enable any shift of the bodyclock, rather than of the exogenous component, to be assessed specifically.

The third possibility is that the change in shape is caused by artefacts of inadequate sampling frequency. This is illustrated by comparing the shapes of Fig. 11.1*a–f*. It is important to realize that the apparent shifts seen in Figs. 11.1*a–f* – and those shifts which can be explained by the other possibilities just described – mean that it is incorrect to assume that they are accurate descriptions of what has happened to the phase of the endogenous component, the bodyclock.

If these difficulties of interpretation cause the cosinor analysis to be used with caution, so too should the comments of DePrins and Waldura (1993). They considered some of the mathematical assumptions made by the cosinor analysis and what happens if they do not hold in a particular case. Briefly, the assumptions are:

(1) the errors in any set of measurements are distributed normally about the predicted values;
(2) there is no serial correlation between the values in the set, that is, the values are independent.

DePrins and Waldura (1993) showed that the parameters estimated by the cosinor analysis are of dubious merit if these assumptions are violated. Unfortunately, it is rarely tested whether or not such assumptions hold. Readers are referred to the original article for more details on how these tests can be carried out.

11.2.4 Alternatives to the single cosine curve

The observation that data often deviate from a sinusoidal rhythm has led to alternative mathematical descriptions of data-spans. Some of these possibilities are outlined below.

One method is to use a model which is a summation of the fundamental period of a cosine curve and various harmonics. For example, periodicities of 6 h, 8 h, 12 h, and so on can be added to the basic cosine curve with its period of 24 h. However, the procedure of adding harmonics to the fundamental period raises a general point with regard to the use of mathematics in biological systems. Increasing mathematical complexity undoubtedly results in the experimental data being better described mathematically; however, the physiological, biochemical, and histological interpretation of such models is often very difficult. There is a very real danger that the biological importance of the rhythm becomes obscured by a complex of mathematical equations.

A different approach which avoids this problem is to consider the biological concepts first and then to base a mathematical model upon them. One example of this would be to describe the value of variable Y at time T, Y_T, as:

$$Y_T = \text{(Endogenous component)}_T$$
$$+ \text{(Exogenous components)}_T + \text{Error}_T \qquad (11.1)$$

The endogenous component is approximated by a cosine curve (see Chapter 1, Fig. 1.1 for the endogenous component during the constant routine). The exogenous component will depend upon the process(es) believed to cause it. Thus, it might be a function of:

(1) time elapsed since last meal (plasma insulin);
(2) time elapsed since last sleep (some forms of mental performance as discussed in Chapter 3);
(3) activity (see exogenous component of Fig. 1.1, obtained by comparing the two curves).

In each case, a mathematical term is required to describe the function. Quadratic or polynomial terms have been used, but a simple yet versatile possibility is:

$$\text{Exogenous component} = B * TE^C$$

where B and C are constants and TE = time elapsed. The value of C determines the general shape of the curve. Thus, with increasing values of TE, the exogenous component:

(1) decreases if $C < 0$;
(2) stays constant if $C = 0$;
(3) increases at a decreasing rate if $0 < C < 1$;
(4) increases linearly if $C = 1$;
(5) increases at an increasing rate if $C > 1$.

The best values for the parameters of the endogenous and exogenous components can then be calculated if data exist which describe the variable (YT) at known times of the day, and after known amounts of time have elapsed since a particular event (TE). The best values will be those that minimize the value of the Error term in eqn. 11.1. This is generally assessed as the sum of the squares of the differences between the data-points and values predicted by the model. The important argument is that the mathematics have been the servant of the biological hypothesis, rather than *vice versa*; there is the advantage that a biological explanation for the results exists *a priori*. Even so, there are some difficulties associated with this approach. These are:

(1) A good mathematical fit to experimental results does not necessarily validate the biological model upon which the equation was based because other models, based on different premises, might fit the data equally well.
(2) It might not always be possible to assess whether one particular set of parameters is statistically significantly better than another.
(3) If the fit to the data is poor, then a change in hypothesis (and type of mathematical function) is required, but the kind of change is not indicated.

Sections 11.2.3 and 11.2.4 and eqn. 11.1 indicate an important problem when the interpretation of results is considered. Since a rhythm consists of endogenous and exogenous components, analyses and interpretations that do not take this into account are limited and might be misleading. That is, fitting a cosine curve to a set of data will not indicate whether changes in the rhythm are due to the endogenous and/or exogenous components of a rhythm. Equations and methods specially designed to assess these components separately are required. The reader is referred to Minors and Waterhouse (1992) for a discussion of some of the possibilities.

11.3 Overview

There are many issues concerned with research design that confront the chronobiologist. They determine the strategy for experimental investigation and how data are collected. Alternative methods of analysing circadian data are available. There is no single method that can be applied to all circadian studies. Analyses and interpretations of data should reflect the existence of endogenous and exogenous components to human circadian rhythms. This applies especially to exercise studies in which exogenous effects are greater than normal.

Further reading

Minors, D. and Waterhouse, J. (1981). *Circadian rhythms and the human*. Wright, Bristol.
Minors, D., and Waterhouse, J. (1988). Mathematical and statistical analysis of circadian rhythms. *Psychoneuroendocrinol.*, **13**, 443–64.
Minors, D. and Waterhouse, J. (1991). Analysis of biological times series. In *Biological rhythms in clinical practice* (ed. J. Arendt, D. Minors, and J. Waterhouse.) pp. 272–93. Bristol, Wright.

References

DePrins, J. and Waldura, J. (1993). Sightseeing around the single cosinor. *Chronobiol. Int.*, **10**, 395–400.

Krieger, D. (1979). Rhythms in CRF, ACTH, and corticosteroids. In *Endocrine rhythms* (ed. D. Krieger), pp. 123–42. Raven Press, New York.

Minors, D. and Waterhouse, J. (1991). Analysis of biological times series. In *Biological rhythms in clinical practice* (ed. J. Arendt, D. Minors, and J. Waterhouse.) pp. 272–93. Bristol, Wright.

Minors, D. and Waterhouse, J. (1992). Investigating the endogenous component of human circadian rhythms: a review of some simple alternatives to constant routines. *Chronobiol. Int.*, **9**, 55–78.

Nelson, W., Tong, U., Lee, J., and Halberg, F. (1979). Methods for cosinor-rhythmometry. *Chronobiologia*, **6**, 305–23.

Index

DATE DUE			
APR 1 0 1998			
OCT 5 1998			
NOV 9 1998			
DEC 15 1998			
GAYLORD			PRINTED IN U.S.A.